Essential Knowledge and Skills for Healthcare Assistants

This revised edition of *Essential Knowledge and Skills for Healthcare Assistants* is an accessible and comprehensive text designed to equip you with the necessary skills for your practice. This book equips you with the knowledge to provide the safest and most effective patient care possible and supplies comprehensive coverage of both primary and secondary care settings, with an emphasis on primary care. It provides evidence-based guidelines to ensure best practice that is matched to the National Occupational Standards, the Care Certificate and the qualification frameworks from around the United Kingdom (UK).

The third edition includes the following:

- an all-new chapter on safeguarding and expanded coverage on communication skills;
- a comprehensive overview of the principal clinical skills that healthcare assistants (HCAs) need to master, including understanding physiological measurements, taking blood pressure, venepuncture, urinalysis, wound care, administering injections, and more;
- essential non-clinical knowledge and skills such as communication and assertiveness, reflection, accountability, confidentiality and record-keeping, health promotion, infection control, and more;
- the evolving role of the healthcare assistant and training opportunities; and
- application to practice throughout, with numerous case studies and activities to aid understanding.

This is an essential guide for all those training as healthcare assistants, nursing associates and assistant practitioners, and a useful reference for students embarking on nursing, and health and social care programmes.

Zoë Rawles BN BSc (Hons) Retired Lecturer/Nurse Practitioner and Director of HealthTrain.

Essential Knowledge and Skills for Healthcare Assistants

Third Edition

Zoë Rawles

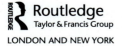

Designed cover credit: Getty Images

Third edition published 2026
by Routledge
4 Park Square, Milton Park, Abingdon, Oxon, OX14 4RN

and by Routledge
605 Third Avenue, New York, NY 10158

Routledge is an imprint of the Taylor & Francis Group, an informa business

© 2026 Zoë Rawles

The right of Zoë Rawles to be identified as author of this work has been asserted in accordance with sections 77 and 78 of the Copyright, Designs and Patents Act 1988.

All rights reserved. No part of this book may be reprinted or reproduced or utilised in any form or by any electronic, mechanical, or other means, now known or hereafter invented, including photocopying and recording, or in any information storage or retrieval system, without permission in writing from the publishers.

Trademark notice: Product or corporate names may be trademarks or registered trademarks, and are used only for identification and explanation without intent to infringe.

First edition published by CRC Press 2014
Second edition published by Routledge 2019

British Library Cataloguing-in-Publication Data
A catalogue record for this book is available from the British Library

ISBN: 978-1-032-60755-9 (hbk)
ISBN: 978-1-032-60624-8 (pbk)
ISBN: 978-1-003-46038-1 (ebk)

DOI: 10.4324/9781003460381

Typeset in Minion Pro
by Apex CoVantage, LLC

This book is for all the amazing healthcare assistants and assistant practitioners I have ever had the privilege to teach or work with, and the many others I have never met.

I hope you find this book useful in your quest for training and knowledge.

Be proud of the wonderful work you do, and keep learning!

Contents

About the author	ix
About the illustrator	xi
Foreword	xiii
Acknowledgements	xv
Glossary	xvii

Introduction	1

Section I: All change — 3

Chapter 1 The evolving role of the healthcare assistant	5

Section II: Some useful stuff — 11

Chapter 2 Understanding reflective practice	13
Chapter 3 Accountability and delegation	23
Chapter 4 Using protocols	29
Chapter 5 Communicating with patients	35
Chapter 6 Simple assertiveness skills	47
Chapter 7 Confidentiality, consent and record-keeping	53
Chapter 8 Safeguarding	65
Chapter 9 Health promotion: the key messages	73
Chapter 10 Keeping it clean: hand decontamination	91
Chapter 11 Chaperoning	101

Section III: Core skills — 109

Chapter 12 Physiological measurements	111
Chapter 13 Understanding and measuring blood pressure accurately	125
Chapter 14 Understanding the heart: how to perform the electrocardiograph (ECG)	135
Chapter 15 Venepuncture and capillary blood testing: best practice	149
Chapter 16 Kidney function and urine: performing accurate urinalysis	167

Section IV: More advanced skills — 175

Chapter 17 Examining the feet of people with diabetes — 177
Chapter 18 The skin and the healing process: basic wound care — 193
Chapter 19 Understanding lung function and disease: performing accurate lung function testing — 209
Chapter 20 Administering immunisations — 223
Chapter 21 Ear irrigation — 253

Index — 267

About the author

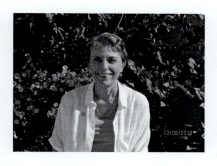

Zoë Rawles qualified as a nurse in 1980, having trained on one of the first nursing degree courses in the country, graduating from the Welsh National School of Medicine in 1980. She spent most of her career working in primary care as a practice nurse. In 1999, she graduated as a nurse practitioner from Swansea University with a first-class honours degree, and subsequently worked as a lecturer on the same course from 2001–2009 during its transition from degree to master's course. In 2010, Zoë co-wrote a book, *Physical Examination Procedures for Advanced Nurses and Independent Prescribers*, with two colleagues. In 2003, while working in general practice, Zoë mentored healthcare assistants who were undergoing training, and she became interested in the developing role of the healthcare assistant. She set up a business (HealthTrain) with a nursing colleague and delivered accredited training for primary care staff, including healthcare assistants. Zoë ran the business single-handedly from 2009–2021, and was instrumental in developing a Level 3 diploma course for HCAs with her local health board (Hywel Dda University Health Board in West Wales).

About the illustrator

Lucy Freegard is an illustrator and children's book author from London. Her books include *Just Like Daddy*, *Just Like Mummy* and *Ballet Bunnies*, published by Pavilion Children's Books. She has an MA in children's book illustration from Cambridge School of Art, a BA in illustration from Cardiff School of Art & Design, and did her Art Foundation at Falmouth University. Lucy lives and works in Bristol.

www.lucyfreegard.com

Foreword

I am delighted to write the foreword for the third edition of *Essential Knowledge and Skills for Healthcare Assistants*. This updated edition is a timely enhancement to the well-received second edition published in 2019.

Healthcare assistants (HCAs) play a crucial role in delivering high-quality care across diverse patient populations, from those in acute settings to individuals with learning disabilities, physical disabilities, mental health conditions and maternity services. As integral members of the healthcare team, HCAs contribute significantly to patient care, and this book is designed to equip them with the essential knowledge and skills necessary for their vital work.

The user-friendly format of this book provides clear guidance and reinforces the importance of patient-centred care throughout. Each chapter is thoroughly researched and written in accessible language, making it an invaluable resource for both new and experienced HCAs. The topics are presented with a combination of step-by-step instructions and real-world insights into the day-to-day experiences of HCAs, particularly in primary care settings. This approach not only aids in understanding responsibilities but also empowers HCAs to practice effectively and with confidence.

Clinical skills form the backbone of the HCA role, and this book excels in detailing these skills with clarity. The addition of a new chapter on safeguarding further enhances its relevance, making it an essential resource for supporting education programmes.

Zoë Rawles, who has been dedicated to the education and training of HCAs since 2003, brings her extensive experience as a former nurse practitioner to this work. Her ability to simplify complex concepts ensures that HCAs can grasp the principles underlying their tasks, gaining the confidence and competence needed for their roles.

This book not only provides the foundational knowledge necessary for current best practices but also addresses essential issues such as accountability, communication, confidentiality and reflection. It is a must-read for anyone aspiring to excel as a healthcare assistant or assistant practitioner, paving the way for safe and effective patient care.

I wholeheartedly recommend *Essential Knowledge and Skills for Healthcare Assistants* as a vital tool for professional development in the healthcare sector.

Ofrah Muflahi, MSc, BSc, SPQ (CCN), RN
Mary Seacole Leadership Scholar '08
RCN UK Professional Lead–Nursing Support Workers

Acknowledgements

My love and sincere thanks to my family, friends and carers who have enabled me to produce this third edition while also caring for my husband who has Alzheimer's.

Glossary

Adjuvant: a substance that is added to a vaccine to increase the body's immune response to the vaccine.

Adrenal insufficiency: a condition whereby the adrenal glands are unable to produce enough steroid hormones such as cortisol. This can be fatal if left untreated.

Alveolus: a tiny air-filled sac at the end of the airways in the lungs. The alveoli are designed to maximise surface area for the exchange of oxygen and carbon dioxide.

Ambulatory blood pressure monitoring: a non-invasive method of recording blood pressure over 24 hours while the patient goes about their normal activities. It is thought to provide an accurate reflection of blood pressure.

Anterolateral: situated in front and to the side.

Anticoagulant: medication that reduces the ability of the blood to clot.

Antibody (also called an immunoglobulin): A protein manufactured by the body that will neutralise a foreign substance or antigen.

Antigen: A substance that will stimulate an immune response by inducing the production of antibodies. An antigen may be a toxin, chemical, bacteria or virus that comes from outside the body.

Anaemia: a condition whereby there are fewer red blood cells or less haemoglobin in each red blood cell. Haemoglobin attaches to oxygen so if there is less of it, the blood is not able to carry as much oxygen around the body.

Anaerobic: living without oxygen.

Aneurysm: a bulge in an artery wall where the wall is weakened and liable to rupture.

Angina: pain that comes from the heart. It occurs when the coronary arteries supplying the heart with blood become narrowed.

Anorexia: lack of appetite.

Anorexia nervosa: an eating disorder characterised by distorted body image and an irrational fear of gaining weight.

Anterior: towards the front.

Antimicrobial: an agent that inhibits the growth of microorganisms or kills them.

Antimuscarinic: the term given to a group of drugs that are smooth muscle relaxants. They will help to dilate or widen the constricted airways in chronic obstructive pulmonary disease (COPD).

Arrythmia: a problem with the rate or rhythm of the heart beat.

Arteriole: a very tiny artery, usually the terminal branch of the artery that connects to the capillary.

Arthropathy: disease of a joint.

Atherosclerosis: a condition whereby the arteries are narrowed by fatty deposits called plaques or atheromas. The restricted blood flow can damage the affected organ (e.g. the heart) and stop it from working properly.

Atrial fibrillation: an abnormal heart rhythm and a major cause of stroke.

Auscultatory: a method of listening to the sounds of the body such as from the heart or lungs, usually using a stethoscope.

Autopsy: examination of a dead body (cadaver) to determine the cause of death.

Axilla: the area under the arm. Also known as the armpit.

Bevel: the sloping point at the sharp end of the needle.

Bilirubin: the yellow pigment in bile produced when the liver breaks down old red blood cells.

Bronchodilator: a substance that dilates (opens up) the airways (bronchi and bronchioles) in the lungs.

Bronchus: the large air tube that begins at the end of the trachea and branches into the lungs.

Bundle of His: a bundle of modified heart muscle that transmits the electrical impulse from the atrio-ventricular node to the right and left ventricles.

Capillary: the smallest blood vessel, where the wall is only one cell thick.

Catalyst: a substance that speeds up a chemical reaction.

Cellulitis: an infection of the deeper layers of the skin usually caused by Group A Streptococcus bacteria.

Glossary

Contraindication: a condition or reason to withhold certain treatment.

Connective tissue: groups of tissue in the body that maintain the form of the body by supporting, anchoring and connecting the various parts of the body.

Cross-contamination: the transfer of a contaminant from one source to another that may result in infection.

Cyanosis: a bluish discoloration of the skin and mucous membranes, usually due to a lack of oxygen in the blood.

Debridement: the removal of dead damaged or infected tissue to enable the healing process.

Deep-vein thrombosis (DVT): the formation of a clot in a deep vein, usually in the leg. If a piece of the clot breaks off and travels to the lung, it can cause a pulmonary embolism, which can be fatal.

Dehydration: a reduction in the normal water content of the body causing an upset in the delicate balance of minerals.

Diaphragm: a sheet of muscle that extends across the bottom of the rib cage separating the thorax from the abdomen.

Domiciliary: provided at home.

Doppler: ultrasound used to examine the blood flow in the major arteries and veins.

Efficacy: the capacity to produce a desired result or effect.

Electrolyte: substances found in the body that carry an electrical charge. They must be present in the right amounts to maintain homeostasis for the proper functioning of the body.

Emphysema: a long-term lung disease whereby there is damage to the air sacs (alveoli) in the lungs.

Endocarditis: inflammation of the inner layer of the heart.

Enzyme: proteins that control the rate of chemical reactions in the body.

Epidemic: a widespread occurrence of an infectious disease occurring in the community during a particular time.

Epithelialisation: migration of newly formed skin cells across a wound bed during the healing process.

Erythrocyte: another name for a red blood cell.

Exacerbation: a worsening or flare-up of symptoms.

Excoriation: tearing or wearing of skin cells, usually due to rubbing or scratching.

Exfoliation: removal of the dead skin cells on the outermost surface of the skin.

Exudates: fluid such as pus or clear fluid leaking out of nearby blood vessels into surrounding tissues or wounds where there is inflammation or infection.

Fistula: an abnormal passage or connection between two organs or areas that do not normally connect. This can result from injury, surgery, infection or inflammation.

Fungating: a type of skin lesion characterised by ulceration and necrosis (death of tissue), usually caused by a cancerous growth breaking through the skin. There is usually a characteristic offensive odour.

Gallipot: a small plastic pot used for holding cleaning fluid, e.g., sodium chloride or water, that may be used during a wound dressing or a minor operation.

Genitourinary tract: the system of organs concerned with the production and excretion of urine and those concerned with reproduction.

Haematological test: a blood test that provides information about the type, number and appearance of red and white blood cells and platelets.

Haematuria: blood in the urine.

Haemoglobin: a substance in red blood cells that combines with and carries oxygen around the body and gives the blood its red colour.

Haemophilia: a hereditary condition whereby the body is unable to control or stop bleeding when a blood vessel is injured.

Heart failure: a condition whereby the heart is unable to pump enough blood to meet the needs of the body.

Hemosiderosis: excessive accumulation of iron deposits called hemosiderin in the tissues.

Hydrophilic: water loving.

Hypercoaguability: a tendency of the blood to coagulate more quickly than normal, increasing the risk of blood clots.

Hypergranulating: where tissue is progressing beyond the surface of the wound in the healing process.

Hyperlipidaemia: a high level of fat (cholesterol, low-density lipoprotein and triglycerides) in the blood. An important risk factor for heart disease.

Hyper-responsiveness (of the airways): a condition whereby the airways in the lungs get smaller (constrict) when exposed to a trigger or allergen.

Hyperthyroidism: a hormonal condition whereby the thyroid gland produces too much thyroxine, which speeds up the body's metabolism.

Hypoallergenic: provokes fewer allergic reactions.

Hypoxia: a deficiency in the amount of oxygen that reaches the tissues of the body.

Immunosuppression: suppression of the body's immune system resulting in an inability to fight infection or disease.

Impermeable: not allowing fluid to pass through.

Inferior vena cava: the large vein that carries deoxygenated blood from the lower half of the body back to the right side of the heart.

In situ: in position.

Insulin resistance: a condition whereby the cells fail to respond to the normal effects of insulin; may progress to Type 2 diabetes.

Intercostal space: the space between two ribs.

Intravenous: within a vein. Usually refers to giving medication or fluid through a tube or needle inserted into the vein.

Ischaemia: reduced blood supply depriving an area of essential oxygen and nutrients.

Ketoacidosis: a complication of diabetes whereby the body is unable to break down glucose because there is not enough insulin. It breaks down fat instead as a source of fuel; this causes the build-up of a by-product called ketones, which can disrupt the body's metabolism.

Leukaemia: cancer of the blood or bone marrow.

Lipoprotein: molecules made of protein and fat that carry cholesterol and similar substances through the blood.

Low adherence: will not stick easily.

Lymph node clearance: removal of lymph nodes from the armpit to check if cancer has spread into the nodes and help determine if further treatment is needed to eliminate any cancerous nodes.

Maceration: a process whereby the skin is softened and broken down by extended exposure to wetness or moisture.

Malaise: a generalised feeling of discomfort or illness; feeling unwell.

Malpractice: negligence or incompetence on the part of a professional.

Metabolic rate: the rate at which the body burns calories.

Mid-clavicular line: an imaginary vertical line crossing through the right or left clavicle (collar bone) to the hip bone.

Mitral valve: a valve made up of a dual flap of skin situated between the left atrium and left ventricle in the heart. It allows blood to flow into the right ventricle when the right atrium contracts but prevents the back flow of blood when the ventricle contracts.

Mucolytic: a medicine that makes sputum less thick and sticky and easier to cough up.

Myocardial infarction: a heart attack resulting from an interruption in the blood supply to an area of heart muscle, causing the heart cells to be damaged or die.

Necrotic: death of cells or tissues through injury or disease where there is an inadequate blood supply. It is irreversible.

Opiate analgesic: a class of drugs derived from the opium poppy that are used to relieve moderate to severe pain.

Orthostatic: related to or caused by standing up.

Palpable: able to be touched or felt.

Palliative: an area of healthcare focused on relieving pain and suffering, to promote quality of life and manage end-of-life symptoms.

Pandemic: an epidemic of an infectious disease across a much larger region, e.g. across continents or even worldwide.

Pathogen: a microorganism capable of causing disease in its host.

Pericardial tamponade: a collection of fluid in the pericardial sac around the heart. It interferes with the performance of the heart and will cause death if left untreated.

Peripheral vascular disease: a condition whereby a build-up of fatty deposits in the arteries restricts the blood supply to the leg muscles.

Pneumothorax: a collection of air in the pleural space around the lungs resulting in collapse of the lung on the affected side.

Polycythaemia: a condition whereby there are too many red blood cells in the blood, resulting in increased thickness or stickiness of the blood reducing blood flow to the organs of the body and sometimes resulting in clots.

Posterior: further back in position.

Postural hypotension: a reduction of at least 20 mm Hg systolic and at least 10 mm Hg diastolic blood pressure within three minutes of standing upright. A common cause of falls in the elderly.

Pre-eclampsia: a medical condition characterised by high blood pressure and protein in the urine that occurs during pregnancy, with risk of serious complications to mother and baby.

Proteinurea: the abnormal presence of protein in the urine in detectable quantities usually defined as an excess of 300 mg protein per day. There are many possible causes but persistent proteinurea should be investigated.

Pulmonary embolism: a blockage in a blood vessel in the lungs which can cause collapse and death.

Pyelonephritis: a kidney infection.

Renal artery stenosis: narrowing of the renal artery (the artery that supplies the kidney with blood) that may lead to impaired kidney function.

Reperfusion: restoration of blood flow after having been blocked.

Sick sinus syndrome: a collection of conditions whereby there is malfunction of the sinus node, resulting in arrhythmia.

Slough: a layer of dead tissue separated from surrounding living tissue that can result in delayed healing. It is made up of dead cells that have accumulated in the exudate and is typically a white/yellow colour.

Statins: a class of drugs used to lower cholesterol.

Sternal border: the long edge of the breast bone.

Superior vena cava: the large vein that carries deoxygenated blood from the upper half of the body back to the right side of the heart.

Supine: lying down with the face up.

Systemic: affecting the entire body.

Thyrotoxicosis: a disease caused by excessive concentrations of thyroid hormones in the body.

Trachea: the large airway that leads from the larynx (voice box) to the bronchi (large airways at the top of the lungs). Also known as the wind pipe.

Tricuspid valve: a three-segmented valve that stops blood in the right ventricle from flowing back into the right atrium.

Turbid: having sediment or particles stirred up or suspended in fluid, clouded, opaque.

Varicose eczema: a type of eczema caused by increased pressure in the veins that affects the legs. Pigment from the blood leaks into the skin, causing discoloration, inflammation and ulceration.

Venuole: a very small blood vessel that allows blood to return from the capillaries to the veins.

Introduction

I was delighted to be asked to write a third edition of this book and for the opportunity to update the information and include an extra chapter on safeguarding.

The first edition was the result of many years of involvement with the training of healthcare assistants (HCAs) and a realisation that most of the books available were aimed more at HCAs working in secondary care. This still appears to be the case, and so for this reason – and because this is the area I know most about – I have once again aimed this book more at HCAs working in primary care. Even so, I hope it will continue to be a useful resource for HCAs and APs working in other areas, as well as for nursing associates and nursing apprentices.

The book covers some of the more theoretical aspects of the role, but also endeavours to provide an accessible and 'user-friendly' approach to learning some of the underpinning knowledge and practical tasks that are now routinely included in the job description of the HCA. It does not assume a level of knowledge, but starts at the grass roots and describes the appropriate skills required for levels 2 and 3 on the career framework outlined by Skills for Health (2010) These are equivalent to GCSE (General Certificate of Secondary Education, grades 4–9) and A levels, respectively. At this level, you – as the HCA or assistant practitioner (AP), also known as associate practitioner – are performing tasks that are delegated to you under supervision from registered professionals. You should always act according to clear protocols and must demonstrate competence supported with the required level of knowledge before being delegated specific tasks.

I have included a chapter on safeguarding in this edition, giving a brief overview of the theory and practical issues involved. There is an example of a safeguarding issue of the sort the HCA may encounter in primary care to get the reader thinking about how they should react in a similar situation.

Whenever possible, the techniques described in this book are based on current national guidelines and are in line with the National Occupational

Essential Knowledge and Skills for Healthcare Assistants

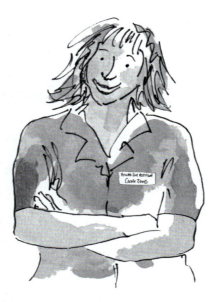

Figure 0.1 Healthcare assistant (female)

Standards (Skills for Health 2023) and referenced accordingly. The book does not replace accredited training, but does provide an essential resource for those currently undergoing such training at levels 2 and 3.

Please read the chapters and engage in the activities and quizzes to reinforce your learning.

I hope you will enjoy developing your understanding about the amazing human body, and discover how you can develop your own essential role in assisting with the monitoring and promotion of health for your patients.

REFERENCES

Skills for Health (2010) *Key Elements of the Career Framework*. http://www.skillsforhealth.org.uk/resources/guidance-documents/163-key-elements-of-the-career-framework (accessed August 7, 2024).

Skills for Health (2023) *National Occupational Standards Overview*. https://www.skillsforhealth.org.uk/resources/national-occupational-standards-overview (accessed August 16, 2024).

Section I
All change

Chapter 1 The evolving role of the healthcare
assistant   5

The evolving role of the healthcare assistant

HEALTHCARE ASSISTANTS AND ASSISTANT PRACTITIONERS

Healthcare assistants are increasingly at the front line of healthcare. There are other titles in use, including healthcare support worker, clinical support worker, nursing support worker and nursing assistant, to name but a few, but for the purposes of this book, I will use the title healthcare assistant (HCA) from here on. The development of the role in recent years, has been exponential and left some nurses shaking their heads in disbelief and asking if their own role is being eroded at a similar rate. Other nurses have embraced the role with open arms, regarding it as an opportunity to develop their own role and broaden their skills in other more complex areas.

It is difficult to establish exactly where and when the HCA role started to enter the scene.

Support workers and HCAs can be found as far back as the Crimean War, and the role of the auxiliary nurse was then established in 1955 (Kessler et al. 2010). The NHS & Community Care Act (1990 Reviewed 2024) formally recognised the HCA role, introducing it as a role to complement the existing auxiliary nursing role. Support workers have since been adopted to a greater or lesser extent in every area of health and social care. The Royal College of Nursing (RCN) has recognised the importance of support workers as providing a large proportion of hands-on care in the many different settings, and describes them as 'the bedrock of our wards, clinics and community teams' (RCN 2024a).

This is quite a leap forward from when I began my nursing career in 1980. I can remember some extraordinarily capable state-enrolled nurses (SENs) and nursing auxiliaries in my early nursing days, but I only became aware of the healthcare assistant role in the mid-1990s. The practice I worked for felt that there was a need for a member of staff to be specifically employed to assist in taking blood pressures and other physiological measurements, as well as performing other various administrative tasks

DOI: 10.4324/9781003460381-3

that were historically part of the practice nurse role. These were considered as tasks that were an inappropriate use of the practice nurse's skills and time. The general practice (GP) contract was also emerging, and practice nurses started to move away from the treatment room and were given responsibility for more chronic disease management. We then needed somebody capable of performing the essential treatment room tasks such as phlebotomy and taking blood pressure. A member of the reception staff was duly sent on the only course for HCAs that was available at the time, and I was asked to be her mentor. This was the start of my long and happy acquaintance with the HCA role. Together with a practice nurse colleague, I became very interested in the emerging role, and we quickly realised that the training provided was either very patchy or non-existent, with little ongoing support for newly trained HCAs. We developed accredited training courses and update days for HCAs, and began to understand the full potential of this new and exciting role in the nursing team.

Other driving forces behind the rise of the HCA role include increasing pressure on primary and secondary healthcare systems due to the ageing population, the rise in chronic disease, advances in medical treatments, increasing costs of delivering healthcare, increasing patient expectations, and shortages of qualified healthcare staff.

The role of AP was developed to plug the gap that existed between the HCAs and registered nurses, and now involves completing or working towards a Level 5 qualification in England and Wales or the equivalent Level 8 qualification in Scotland, e.g. Diploma of Higher Education, Foundation Degree, Higher National Diploma or NVQ Level 5. The AP is described as working at a higher level than the HCA with a more in-depth understanding of the factors that influence health and ill health (RCN 2024b)

WHAT IS HAPPENING ABOUT REGULATION?

When I wrote each previous edition of this book, I assumed that at some stage, HCAs and APs would be regulated and that there would be some sort of pathway into nurse training for APs. Bearing in mind the complexity of some of the tasks performed it seemed a logical conclusion to me. However, here we are – yet another four years on – and still there is no regulation of HCAs and APs. So as before, anyone can put on a badge that states 'Healthcare Assistant' and no one is any the wiser in terms of how much or how little training that individual has had. Regulation would eliminate this scandalous anomaly, and would result in standardised training, competencies and conduct for the HCA/AP, and a clearer understanding of the role for all concerned, thereby ensuring safer practice and improving the outcome for the worker, the employer and, most importantly, the patient. In 2013, the call for regulation was given a huge boost with the publication of the Report of the Mid Staffordshire NHS Foundation Trust (2013). The inquiry was set up following the disclosure of appalling care resulting in patient suffering, and in many cases premature death, in hospitals within the Mid Staffordshire NHS Foundation Trust. The report made many recommendations, including the need for a uniform description of healthcare support workers that clearly distinguished them from registered nurses. It also recommended that healthcare support workers working for the NHS or for the independent sector should be registered and have a national code of conduct, with a common set of national standards for education and training to be overseen by the Nursing and Midwifery Council (NMC). We do now at least have codes of conduct for healthcare support workers (HCSWs), and most Foundation Trusts and Health Boards are now striving to make some sort of training mandatory as far as possible. In my local Health Board of Hywel Dda, we set up and delivered an accredited Level 3 diploma course over 12 months which was part of an all-Wales initiative, free to all HCAs working in primary care and specifically designed for their needs. There has also been the Care Certificate that was launched in England in 2015 by skillsforcare.org.uk (Skills for Care 2015) which attempted to introduce a form of voluntary induction training for HCAs. It identifies a set of standards that HCAs should adhere to in their daily working life, specifically in areas such as role development, communication skills, patient dignity and privacy. Uptake remains variable, however, with many appearing to be unaware of its existence. Hopefully this will improve, and it is certainly a step in the right direction, but because these innovations are very dependent on voluntary participation, uptake of the training will always be an issue. I feel very strongly that regulation is the real issue here, but we are sadly no closer to this now than we were ten years ago. This is hugely disappointing, and I wonder what catastrophe will have to happen before this is addressed. Until regulation for HCAs and APs happens, they must be given every opportunity and be actively encouraged to attend relevant courses and achieve accredited training to ensure competence in their area of work. It should not be acceptable for the ideology of 'see one, do one' to apply to HCAs or APs, whose range of ability and knowledge can vary so hugely. The public (you and me!) have a right to expect that when they are treated by a healthcare worker, that person has the relevant training and competence.

WHAT ABOUT NURSING ASSOCIATES AND NURSING APPRENTICES?

In the second edition of this book, I wrote about the new healthcare role of the nursing associate (NA) and trainee nursing associate (TNA) that were introduced by the Department of Health in England in 2017. As with the AP role, they were introduced to bridge the gap between HCAs and registered nurses, but for this group, there is now a recognised route into nursing for those who want to make that career move. Understandably, there continue to be concerns voiced by APs who wonder where their role will fit in the grand scheme of things. Hopefully there will be some sort of bridging programme to allow APs to become NAs, but this has yet to be clarified. The good news is that at least the NAs are now regulated by the NMC.

At present, the NA role has only been introduced in England, and there are no immediate plans to introduce them in Northern Ireland, Scotland or Wales. I think there is a legitimate concern that the distinction between RNs and registered NAs is too much of a grey area and is not the answer to the shortage of nurses in the NHS. This role is not the same as the nursing apprentice, which enables people to train to become a graduate registered nurse through an apprentice route and is therefore is a new direct route into nursing, whereby students may work as HCAs (Figure 1.1) while also completing their degree-level training over at least four years.

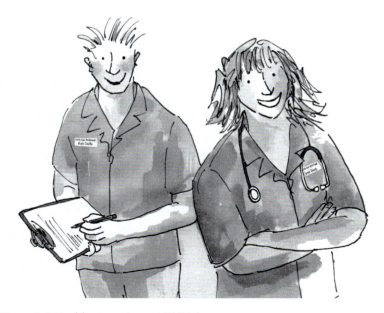

Figure 1.1 Healthcare assistants (HCAs)

Confused? Yes, me, too – still confused after ten years! I have tried to summarise the situation as it pertains to primary care in what follows, but unfortunately it seems to have become unnecessarily complicated.

HCA – not regulated or registered but voluntary training encouraged. Care Certificate suggests required standards. No direct route into nurse training.

AP – not regulated or registered but training required at Level 5 (England and Wales) and Level 8 (Scotland). No direct route into nurse training.

Trainee Nurse Associate + Nurse Associate (England only at present) – registered and regulated by NMC with recognised route into nurse training. Will work towards Level 5 qualification but can also work towards Level 6 nursing apprentice degree.

Nursing Apprentice – will work towards a Level 6 nursing degree to become an RN.

REFERENCES

Kessler, I., Heron, P., Dopson, S. et al. (2010) *The Nature and Consequences of Support Workers in a Hospital Setting: Final Report.* London: NHS Institute for Health. https://www.researchgate.net/publication/229049129 (accessed August 2, 2024).

NHS & Community Care Act 1990 (Reviewed 2024). http://www.legislation.gov.uk/ukpga/1990/19/contents (accessed August 29, 2024).

Report of the Mid Staffordshire NHS Foundation Trust Public Inquiry (2013). https://assets.publishing.service.gov.uk/media/5a7ba0faed915d13110607c8/0947.pdf (accessed October 21, 2024).

RCN (2024a) *Nursing Support Workers.* https://www.rcn.org.uk/Professional-Development/Nursing-Support-Workers (accessed August 2, 2024).

RCN (2024b) *Assistant Practitioner.* https://www.rcn.org.uk/Professional-Development/Your-career/HCA/Assistant-Practitioner (accessed October 21, 2024).

Skills for Care (2015) *Care Certificate.* https://www.skillsforcare.org.uk/Developing-your-workforce/Care-Certificate/Care-Certificate.aspx (accessed August 7, 2024).

Section II
Some useful stuff

Chapter 2	Understanding reflective practice	13
Chapter 3	Accountability and delegation	23
Chapter 4	Using protocols	29
Chapter 5	Communicating with patients	35
Chapter 6	Simple assertiveness skills	47
Chapter 7	Confidentiality, consent and record-keeping	53
Chapter 8	Safeguarding	65
Chapter 9	Health promotion: the key messages	73
Chapter 10	Keeping it clean: hand decontamination	91
Chapter 11	Chaperoning	101

Understanding reflective practice

2

WHAT IS REFLECTION AND WHAT IS THE POINT?

What happens when something goes wrong in work? Suppose, for example, that you take a blood sample but forget to label it, or a patient becomes angry and hostile after being kept waiting, or a colleague is critical of your work, or you are asked to do something that you feel is out of your sphere of competence. The list is endless, and I suspect many of you reading this will recognise at least one of the examples given. So, what do you do about it when it happens? Think about it for a while, then forget about it until it happens again? Chat about it over a cup of coffee with a friend who is on your side and is very reassuring? Carry on with your busy clinic and think of it as 'one of those things'? Or maybe it stays on your mind for a bit longer, at least until you get home, when it gets pushed to the bottom of the priority list, competing against collecting the children from school or deciding what to cook for tea. If this is what happens, then the chances are it wasn't a very useful learning experience, and as a result it is more likely to happen again.

Alternatively, and just as importantly, you will have some very good experiences, such as a clinic that goes particularly well or positive feedback on your work from colleagues or patients. You need to learn from all these various experiences and can only do this if you can establish the factors that contributed to the outcome of that practice. Depending on whether the outcome was good or bad, you can then endeavour to change your practice or try to repeat it in the future.

Sometimes it is also useful to question established and accepted practice to determine if that is the best way of doing something and consider if or how it could be improved.

Reflection is the process we can use to look back on our work, and although it is usually thought of as a tool to learn from mistakes or poor practice, I hope you will discover that it can be so much more than this.

DOI: 10.4324/9781003460381-5

HOW CAN WE LEARN FROM OUR EXPERIENCES?

This is where a structured reflective process can be a useful tool, and one worth developing and nurturing as you hurtle through your busy working life. If you can learn to reflect honestly and thoroughly on your work and experiences, you will ultimately become a safer practitioner, protecting yourself and your patients. Your job satisfaction is likely to improve as well.

Reflective practice can enable us to do the following.

- Study our own decision-making processes.
- Be constructively critical of our relationship with our colleagues.
- Analyse hesitations and skill and knowledge gaps.
- Face problematic and painful episodes.
- Identify learning needs.

(Bolton 2014)

Reflection is a strategy to develop learning and understanding through experience. It allows the practitioner to understand the experience differently and move on to provide safer practice, less likely to repeat past mistakes. Reflection involves consciously thinking about the experience (as opposed to mulling it over for a few minutes) and actively making decisions. It does not need to be intrusive or time-consuming, and neither should the potential complexity of the skills involved be viewed as a barrier to the process. It can be as simple or as complicated as you want it to be. Reflection is thought to be a way of bridging the theory/practice gap (Bulman and Schutz 2004), and it is important to enable us to transfer learning into practice (Chapman and Law 2009).

Writing the reflection down is especially useful (see Figure 2.1), and it can help the process by allowing the writer to effectively freeze the film, reflect on it, rewind and review a previous scene having reflected upon a later one (Bolton 2014). Jasper (2003) suggests that the process of writing things down enables us to unlock secrets that have puzzled us or learn things about ourselves and those around us. It is a way of discovering more about yourself and your subject (Bolton 2014). When appropriate, written records might then be discussed with a trusted supervisor so that you can share your collective experience to make sense of the challenges encountered.

Understanding reflective practice

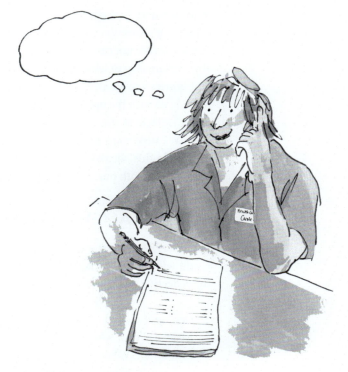

Figure 2.1 Reflecting on practice

SO, WHAT DO YOU WRITE ABOUT AND HOW DO YOU WRITE IT?

Even for nurses with many years of experience, the process of writing meaningful reflection can still be a daunting task. Part of the problem lies in the fact that at times it can be an uncomfortable experience. You might begin to realise that what happened occurred as a direct result of your action, what you did and how you behaved. Jasper (2003) suggests that this is a very mature way of learning, to be able to revisit and take responsibility for actions and choices, but for this to occur you need to be self-aware and have considerable insight into your behaviour, and this can take time to develop. Writing the reflection down also becomes a way of 'knowing' and a method of discovery and analysis (Bolton 2014).

Compiling a reflective diary is a good starting place for those of you who are new to reflective writing. There are also many frameworks or tools that have been developed to assist in the art of structured written reflection, and they may help as a reminder of the different dimensions of reflection and dissuade us from focusing on only that which seems comfortable or convenient. We are all good at telling stories, but all too often, our stories are uncritical and self-protective, providing us with an acceptable explanation of what happened to make us feel better about ourselves. Our stories are an attempt to create order out of chaos, but they rarely provide us with the opportunity to develop as people. To do this, we need to try to look at the story from a different and maybe strange point of view. We need to re-examine the story from a different perspective. If we cannot do this, we risk only ever seeing the world from our own limited view, in line with our own 'truth'.

SOME FRAMEWORKS FOR REFLECTION

Gibbs' (1988) *reflective cycle* is one of the older models, but nevertheless is still widely used today. Gibbs describes the following six key stages in the reflective process.

1 *Description* of what happened.
2 *Feelings*: What were you thinking and feeling?
3 *Evaluation*: What was good and what was bad about the experience?
4 *Analysis*: What sense can you make of the situation?
5 *Conclusion*: What else could you have done?
6 *Action plan*: What will you do next time?

Driscoll (2007) provides an alternative framework with the following three simple stages.

1 *What?* What happened?
2 *So what?* The analysis. How did it make you feel or how do you think the others involved felt, and why is it important?
3 *Now what?* Action plan. What do you do next?

Oelofsen (2012) provides a three-step process designated as follows.

1 *Curiosity*: Why do we do things in certain ways? What is my contribution? Is there anything for me to learn from my own actions?
2 *Looking closer*: A journey towards understanding. Taking a closer look at the event to reflect on according to the questions produced in step 1. Remember, though, that there are not always clear answers to questions, but they may provide us with the impetus to find out more.

3 *Transformation*: A journey towards action, using the understanding gained and starting to implement new ideas. This stage is about enhancing personal competence and improving service.

The *REFLECT model* (Barksby et al. 2015) is a more recent addition to the reflection frameworks, and is a modification of the Gibbs (1988) framework whereby the word 'REFLECT' has been used as a mnemonic to make the steps in the process easier to remember. This model describes the following seven essential steps.

1 R: *Recall* the events.
2 E: *Examine* your responses.
3 F: Acknowledge *feelings*.
4 L: *Learn* from the experience.
5 E: *Explore* options.
6 C: *Create* a plan of action.
7 T: Set *timescale*.

None of these models are perfect, and sometimes it is very difficult to fit the story under the headings. Don't get bogged down by this. It does help to have some sort of structure, but if your story won't fit under the headings, then make up another heading!

EXAMPLE OF A REFLECTIVE ACCOUNT

The following account is an example of what I feel was a very good reflection. It was presented to me as part of a portfolio that an HCA student on one of my courses had to complete. I had her permission to recreate her account here, but I am unable to credit her with this as she opted for anonymity. She chose to use Gibbs' reflective cycle for her reflection.

Describe what happened

I was asked to chaperone a locum doctor while he performed a breast examination. I had not had any chaperone training and was unsure of what to do or where to stand, so I stood quite awkwardly at the foot of the bed while he carefully examined both breasts. The doctor was unable to feel any lump, although the lady was quite sure she had felt a lump in her right breast. He then asked me to feel the breasts to see if I could feel anything. I was surprised and alarmed at his request, but thought I should try, as he was the doctor and I didn't feel able to say no to his request. I have never been trained to examine breasts, so I had no idea how to do it and felt very embarrassed doing it. I think the patient could feel my embarrassment, and she herself seemed surprised that he had asked me to do it. She tried to point to where she could feel the lump, but I was unable to feel anything. The doctor then thanked me for my help and told the lady to redress, at which point I left the room.

I was worried about this, but thought I might be making more of it than I needed to. Nevertheless, the next day I discussed it with my practice nurse, and together we went to see the practice manager and explained the situation to her. She also felt that the doctor should not have asked me to do the examination. The senior partner (Dr A) came into the room when we were talking, and he got involved, too. He was very shocked that I had been asked to do this. The locum doctor in question had only been employed on that one occasion and was unlikely to be employed by them again, but Dr A felt there should be something in place to prevent this sort of situation from arising again. Everybody was very supportive and understood why I didn't feel able to say no, but reassured me that in future if I was not happy to do something, I should say so, and that they would always support me in this, regardless of who had asked me to do it.

Dr A suggested a list of surgery staff with their job roles/responsibilities be given to each locum/new member of staff so that everybody would understand each other's roles, and it would be easier to say no if a task you were being asked to do was not covered in your job description.

We also discussed the issue of chaperoning, and I explained that I was unsure of what I was doing. It seemed as if a lot of non-clinical members of staff had also raised concerns about this to the practice manager, and she had arranged some training for us, so hopefully in future I will feel more comfortable with this role.

What were my feelings?

Initially, I felt very awkward standing and watching the breast examination. I didn't know where to stand or where to look, so I looked the other way so I didn't add to the lady's embarrassment. When the doctor then asked me to examine the breasts, I didn't feel I could say no, so although I had no idea how to do it, I carried on and did the best I could. I felt that the doctor must want a second opinion and was confident in my ability to help him. This was quite flattering, but I didn't want to do it and felt very uncomfortable. I wished I had felt strong enough to say no. I didn't feel that he should have asked me to do this, and I don't think the lady was happy about it, either. I did ask her if she was OK with me checking, but I don't think she felt she could say no either, so it didn't feel as if I was having proper informed consent, and this worried me.

When I spoke to my practice nurse about this afterwards, she was horrified that the doctor had asked me to do this, and was quite adamant that I should have refused, but understood why I found it difficult.

I did feel very happy that everyone was very supportive and not at all dismissive, as I had thought they might be.

Evaluation: What was good and bad about the experience?

This situation was very difficult for me because of the following.

Bad points

- The locum doctor put me in an awkward situation by asking me to do something I was not trained to do.
- I felt unable to say no, and if I am honest, I was a little bit flattered that he had enough confidence in me to ask me to do it, so I agreed to do something that I was not comfortable with, which compromised patient safety.
- I did not have proper informed consent, so I infringed the patient's rights and I was open to accusations of abuse from the patient.
- The patient might have been falsely reassured that she had no lump in her breast.
- I did not understand my role as chaperone and felt awkward doing this.
- I was unsure about what to do and felt as though I might be making an unnecessary fuss.

Good points

- I did do something about this because I knew it felt wrong.
- I felt that I could discuss it with my senior nurse colleague and practice manager.

- I learnt a lot from this experience, namely that it is OK to say no to something, even if it is a doctor who is asking me, and that my colleagues in the surgery will always support me if my refusal is reasonable.
- In future, all new members of staff will be informed about what each person can and can't do, so there should be no more misunderstandings.
- We will all have chaperone training, so will feel more confident about how to do this properly.

Analysis: What sense can I make from it?

The Code of Conduct for Healthcare Support Workers in England (Skills for Health 2013) includes the following guidance, and I feel that on this occasion I failed to deliver on all these points:

1 Be accountable for your actions or omission.
2 Promote and uphold the privacy, dignity, rights, health and well-being of people who use the health service.
3 Work in collaboration with your colleagues to ensure delivery of high-quality, safe and compassionate healthcare, care and support.
4 Communicate in an open and effective way to promote the health, safety and well-being of people who use healthcare services.

Conclusion

Looking back on this incident, I feel very glad I did do something about this because it would have been easy to just forget about it and put it down to a bad experience. If I had done this, I would have no clear idea of what to do should the situation arise again, and I would probably end up making the same mistakes.

After discussing things with my nurse mentor, practice manager and Dr A, I know that I must always say no to anything I feel uncomfortable about doing. I may need to develop some confidence to do this, but knowing that my colleagues will support me is very helpful.

I also realise that I am uncomfortable chaperoning and that I need to address this.

Reflecting on this incident has been very useful because it has helped me to learn from it, and it has reinforced how this will change my practice in the future. It has also resulted in some very positive changes for the practice generally.

I also feel now that I will be able to follow the code of conduct to ensure the safety and well-being of my patients.

Action plan

In the future, I will always say no if asked to do anything that is 'out of my comfort zone' or that I have not been trained to do. I will try to develop some assertive skills by doing some research online and will also attend any relevant training there may be on this. I will always go to my nurse or manager if I have any problems such as this again. I will also attend the chaperone training that is to be provided in the surgery so that I feel more confident about my role as chaperone.

ACTIVITY

Try to restructure the reflection provided using one of the other frameworks. See if you can work out which bits of the reflection fit under the headings provided by Gibbs (1988) and Oelofsen (2012).

Now have a go at a reflection yourself using whichever framework you find the easiest to work with. You can even use a mixture of them, but make sure that you have some structure to your reflection so that you avoid waffling and getting nowhere. Be honest about your feelings and how you think others may have felt. Your reflection can be about anything – big or small – that happened to you in work, and it can be about something that went well or badly. It may be something you still found yourself thinking about at the end of a busy day, but remember to keep it simple to begin with. It doesn't have to be as lengthy as the example – sometimes very brief reflections can be just as useful!

I hope you will find reflection useful and that you will continue to use and develop this skill in the future. Throughout the book, there will be more opportunities for you to practise some structured reflection. Be sure to have a go!

You might also want to check out Chapter 6 on assertiveness skills and Chapter 11 on chaperoning if the reflective account raised any issues for you.

REFERENCES

Barksby, J., Butcher, N., and Whysall, A. (2015) A new model of reflection for clinical practice. *Nursing Times* 111(34/35): 21–23. https://www.nursingtimes.net/Journals/2015/08/15/t/e/e/190815_A-new-model-of-reflection-for-clinical-practice.pdf (accessed August 7, 2024).

Bolton, G. (2014) *Reflective Practice. Writing and Professional Development* (4th ed). SAGE Publications Ltd.

Bulman, C., and Schutz, S. (eds) (2004) *Reflective Practice in Nursing*. Oxford: Blackwell Scientific Publications.

Chapman, A., and Law, S. (2009) Bridging the gap: An innovative dementia learning program for health care assistants in hospital wards using facilitator-led discussions. *International Psychogeriatrics* 21(Suppl. 1): S58–S63. https://www.ncbi.nlm.nih.gov/pubmed/19288962 (accessed October 21, 2024).

Driscoll, J. (2007) *Practising Clinical Supervision: A Reflective Approach for Healthcare Professionals* (2nd ed). Balliere Tindall Elsevier.

Gibbs, G. (1988) *Learning by Doing: A Guide to Teaching and Learning*. London: Further Educational Unit.

Jasper, M. (2003) *Beginning Reflective Practice*. Cheltenham: Nelson Thornes Ltd.

Oelofsen, N. (2012) *Developing Reflective Practice: A Guide for Students and Practitioners of Health and Social Care*. Oxford: Scion.

Skills for Health (2013) *Code of Conduct for Healthcare Support Workers and Adult Social Care Workers*. http://www.skillsforhealth.org.uk/standards/item/217-code-of-conduct (accessed August 2, 2024).

Accountability and delegation

In your role as HCA, you will constantly be asked to accept and perform tasks that have been delegated to you by the registered nurse or doctor. It is vital that you and the person delegating the task to you understand the individual roles in the process of delegation and what exactly each of you is accountable for.

When I first started delivering training for HCAs, I had many long, interesting and sometimes heated discussions with registered nurses who were understandably anxious about being held accountable for the actions of the HCA. Since then, HCAs have become so much a part of the team in most areas that I think nurses are more aware of the issues. It can, however, still be a controversial area, with some grey areas that are not always easy to resolve. In this chapter, there will be an attempt to explore and clarify some of the main issues.

DEFINING ACCOUNTABILITY

When you are accountable, you are personally responsible for the outcome or the consequences of your actions. There are various types of accountability, including the following.

- *Legal accountability*: This is the obligation of every citizen to obey the laws of the country. In addition to this, the law imposes a 'duty of care' on all health workers (including HCAs, APs, NAs, students, registered nurses and doctors) when it is possible that they might cause harm to their patients through their actions or failure to act (Cox 2010).
- *Professional accountability*: This is the additional obligation of the professional not to abuse trust and to be able to justify professional actions.

Prerequisites for accountability:

- *Responsibility*: Job description, standards, protocols.
- *Authority*: Appropriate registration, training, qualification.
- *Ability*: Knowledge and skills to perform the activity.

Responsibility and authority require knowledge and the ability to understand the alternatives, reasons and consequences of a decision.

The NMC's 'The Code' (NMC 2024) advises that registrants (i.e., registered nurses) should only delegate tasks and duties that are within the other person's scope of competence and ensure that the other person understands the instructions they are given. The registrant should also provide adequate support and supervision, and be able to confirm that outcomes of delegated tasks meet the required standards. Obviously, the registered nurse cannot perform every intervention for every patient, so they will need to delegate some tasks, and in this instance, they become accountable for the appropriate delegation of the task.

There is very little guidance regarding which activities can or cannot be delegated; this has meant that in some areas, HCAs are performing quite complex tasks, while in others, they are not allowed to do much at all. A good example that is still creating much debate in various areas of the UK is that of ear irrigation. Some local authorities have decided that HCAs should never be allowed to perform irrigation, while others have embraced it as a task very suitable for competent HCAs, providing that they have had suitable training and have appropriate supervision in place. Incidentally, ear irrigation is also controversial for other reasons at the time of writing this, as discussed in Chapter 21.

DELEGATION

Questions to consider when a task is delegated to an HCA include the following.

- Is this in the *best interests of the patient*?
- Does it involve *clinical risk*, and if so, is the risk significant?
- Who has the *authority and appropriate clinical knowledge* to agree that this task can be delegated?
- Is the *person delegating the task competent* in it themselves?
- Is the *HCA competent* in the task to be delegated, with written evidence of their competence, preferably in line with recognised standards such as the National Occupational Standards (Skills for Health 2023)?
- Will it be *beneficial to the HCA role*, and do they have the capacity to take it on?

Having considered these points and decided to proceed with the delegation, there are some basic rules that should be followed to ensure that both the person delegating the task and the HCA are protected, and that patient care and safety is not compromised in any way.

Be *clear about the task* to be delegated and have clear *ground rules*. Check that the *job description* includes the new task, and make sure there are robust procedures or *protocols* in place. These protocols must be regularly reviewed and should specify *when the HCA should seek further advice*. Be sure there is *appropriate insurance cover* for the new task.

Check that *all members of the team are aware of the new task* and the restrictions. Negotiate time for regular *supervision and support*, and ensure there is access to regular *updates* at appropriate intervals.

There are some useful resources online for induction and as an adjunct to training. The RCN First Steps website is one such resource RCN (2022).

Finally, any new task should be *evaluated* after an appropriate amount of time to assess the impact on all concerned.

HCAs remain unregulated at the time of writing this edition (2024), so each case will have to be assessed individually, and some will be more willing and able to take on the various tasks than others.

At the heart of this is the undisputed fact that the registered nurse or the doctor is accountable for the *appropriateness of the delegation*. In some cases, nurses have found themselves in a position where they disagree with a nurse or doctor colleague on the appropriateness of delegation to the HCA. In this instance, they should make it clear from the outset that they will not be held accountable for the delegation, and should put this in writing.

So where do *you* – as the HCA – fit in all of this? If you accept a task, are you accountable? As an HCA, you don't have a professional body such as the NMC in the way that nurses do, but *you are still accountable to yourself, your employer, your delegating nurse and – most importantly – your patient*. So, if you feel as if you have been delegated a task for which you have not had appropriate training or whenever you are in any doubt about your competence, you should always say no until you have had further advice or clarification.

Check out Chapter 6 on assertiveness skills if you have problems saying no.

ACTIVITY

Now have a look at the following scenario and see how you get on.

Scenario: a complicated dressing – who is accountable?

You are working alone as the nurse is off sick and a patient comes in for a dressing change. They have an open wound that requires packing with ribbon gauze to avoid the wound healing over the top too quickly. You have never done this type of

Essential Knowledge and Skills for Healthcare Assistants

dressing before, and are not sure if you should go ahead and do it, but the patient is insistent, as they are unable to get to the local hospital, which is some distance away, to have the dressing done, and it really needs doing today. You ring the doctor and check with him. He is busy with another patient, and says you will just have to do the best you can.

What will you do?

If you decide to go ahead, who is accountable if something goes wrong?

Suggested answers are in Box 3.1.

Box 3.1 Suggested answers to the 'a complicated dressing' scenario

You should not agree to do this, even though the doctor has effectively given you permission to do so. You know you are not competent to perform this type of dressing and are not sure that the doctor would know how to do it, either. There is no protocol to guide you for this, and there is no care plan in place. You must be assertive enough to say no and find another way of helping instead. Perhaps you could book some transport for the patient to get to the hospital or prepare the equipment for the doctor to do the dressing instead.

If you agree to go ahead and there is a problem afterwards, you will be accountable for accepting a task that you are not competent to do. You could be accused of negligence, although ultimately, the GP would have to accept vicarious liability for this.

Accountability and delegation

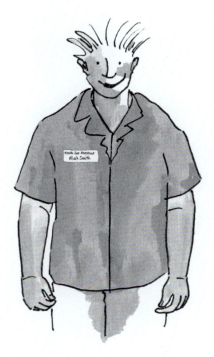

Figure 3.1 HCA (male)

REFERENCES

Cox, C. (2010) Legal responsibility and accountability. *Nursing Management* 17(3): 18–20.

NMC (2024) *The Code.* https://www.nmc.org.uk/standards/code (accessed September 7, 2024).

RCN (2022) *First Steps.* https://rcnlearn.rcn.org.uk/Search/RCN-First-Steps (accessed September 2, 2024).

Skills for Health (2023) *National Occupational Standards Overview.* https://www.skillsforhealth.org.uk/resources/national-occupational-standards-overview (accessed August 16, 2024).

Using protocols

Throughout this book, you will see many references to procedures and *protocols*. You may wonder what protocols are and why they are so important. This chapter will discuss the issue of protocols in practice and provide a basic template for a protocol. I have used the word *protocols* in the chapter title, as this is the term most nurses and HCAs are familiar with, but you may also use the term *clinical guidelines*, and the two terms will be used interchangeably.

For HCAs who perform nursing duties that have been delegated by a nurse and for the nurses who are delegating the care, there must be clear protocols in place to protect both parties and to ensure good quality care for the patient. Without written protocols in place, you may unwittingly be performing tasks that are inappropriate for your role or competence. You may also be making clinical judgements or decisions that ultimately result in unsafe practice.

Care Quality Commission (CQC) inspectors (in England) will want to see that practices have robust systems in place to ensure patients receive safe, high-quality care during an inspection. Practice procedures and protocols will be key to their assessment of this (CQC 2022; Skills for Care 2022).

THE PURPOSE OF A PROTOCOL

The protocol should be clear and unambiguous, stating the actions to be taken and the reason for those actions. This should enable the HCA to take the action most likely to result in the best possible outcome for the patient and reduce the risk of any problems.

Protocols or guidelines exist at national and local levels. At the national level, we have guidelines created by the National Institute for Health and Clinical Excellence (NICE) and other healthcare organisations, such as the British Heart Foundation, the British Hypertension Society, the

DOI: 10.4324/9781003460381-7

Royal College of Nursing and the British Thoracic Society. At the local level, guidelines can be produced by trusts, at ward level or within general practice. A nurse or HCA may be working within national *and* local guidelines.

In this chapter, we will just consider local protocols or guidelines developed in the work setting. They can include the actual procedure, but should also include information about who is able to perform the procedure, the training required, the patient group with inclusion and exclusion criteria, materials to be used for the procedure, referral guidelines, review dates and signatures of all the healthcare workers involved. They should always be based on current national guidelines, current available evidence or expert consensus, and they should usually be reviewed annually. They may be reviewed sooner if the evidence or national guidelines change. Good clinical guidelines should:

- provide a clear outline of the purpose and scope of the document;
- be clear and well presented; and
- be applicable to practice.

Clinical guidelines or protocols are advisory only, and should never be used without assessing the specific patient or situation first. Depending on the patient's condition, you may decide it is inappropriate to use the protocol. If for any reason the protocol is not followed, the full reason for this, with information about the alternative course of action that was taken, should be documented. *Always seek advice from the registered nurse or doctor if you are unsure about anything.*

Protocols should not be kept in a drawer gathering dust. Make sure you read them and know what they include – and then use them!

In each chapter on clinical skills in this book, the procedure for the task has been provided, and is always based on current evidence or national guidelines. You may want to use these in protocols that you develop with your nurse, but you should also include other information, as discussed previously.

Initially, the plan for this chapter was to provide a protocol for every clinical procedure outlined in this book. However, it felt more useful to have the guidance for the procedure outlined in the relevant chapters, so instead I have produced a template that you can adapt for each clinical procedure by inserting the step-by-step procedure in the appropriate place as indicated.

> Remember, if a guideline exists and the nurse (or HCA) has failed to follow it, this may be considered in a court of law when deciding if the legal duty of care has been breached (Tingle and McHale 2007).

A PROTOCOL TEMPLATE FOR AN HCA WORKING IN GENERAL PRACTICE (USING DIABETIC FOOT EXAMINATION AS AN EXAMPLE)

Name of surgery: ....

This guideline is written to enable HCAs that have received appropriate training in adult diabetic foot assessment and have been assessed as competent by their mentor (name: . . . .) to perform a diabetic foot assessment, prior to the patient's attendance in clinic with the GP or diabetic nurse. It may sometimes be necessary to perform foot assessment clinics at other times, as well, but in this instance, if the HCA has any concerns about the condition of the feet, they must ask their registered nurse mentor or GP to check before the patient leaves the surgery.

The HCA will document each foot assessment on the computer notes using the diabetic template. They will also note the interval before the next assessment.

Inclusion criteria

Patients aged 18 or older who are under the care of the surgery for their diabetes.

Exclusion criteria

Children under the age of 18.

Patients with complex health needs (as decided by GP).

Patients with a history of active foot ulceration or amputation.

Procedure

Insert procedure guidelines here (see Chapter 17).

Classify the risk of ulceration and refer appropriately

Insert information about risk assessment here (see Chapter 17).

Advice and follow-up

Patient to be provided with appropriate leaflet on foot care (such as one from Diabetes UK).

HCA to ensure patient understands the importance of reporting *any* problems immediately.

Reporting concerns

When the HCA is in *any* doubt about any aspect of the foot examination, they must always ensure that the GP/diabetic nurse is made aware and inspects the patient's feet.

Signed (GP) . . . . Signed (nurse mentor) . . . .

Signed (HCA) . . . .

Date . . . . Review date . . . .

References

Insert references for any information used in the protocol here.

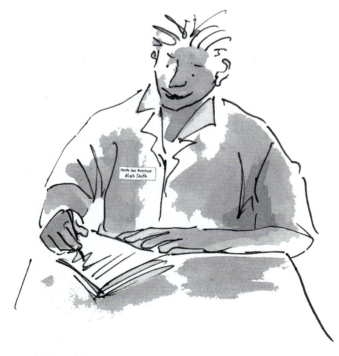

Figure 4.1 HCA writing

Box 4.1 Case study: working without a protocol

Joe the HCA (level 3) was taking a blood pressure (BP) reading. He had no protocol to work to, but considered himself to be competent in the task. A patient attended for a blood pressure check and his blood pressure was 170/102. Joe had no protocol, and the doctor and nurse were both busy, so he didn't want to bother them. He thought it seemed reasonable to recheck the patient's BP in one month. When the patient returned a month later, his BP was 220/130 and he was admitted to hospital. The GP told Joe he should have referred the patient to him on the same day.

In this instance, Joe had made a clinical judgement based on inadequate knowledge and training. He did not have a protocol, so when in doubt, he had to make these decisions himself or constantly refer to the nurse or GP for advice. The protocol for blood pressure monitoring should clearly state the correct procedure, as well as the parameters for action, including monitoring intervals and when to refer to the nurse or GP. This ensures that the HCA is never put in a position where they make a clinical decision. In a court of law, Joe could be held accountable for making a clinical decision for which he was not qualified. The nurse who delegated the task could also be held accountable, and both the HCA and the nurse could be accused of negligence. The GP employer would then accept liability under the vicarious liability principle.

REFERENCES

CQC (2022) *Health Care Assistants in General Practice*. https://www.cqc.org.uk/guidance-providers/gps/gp-mythbusters/gp-mythbuster-57-health-care-assistants-general-practice (accessed August 16, 2024).

Skills for Care (2022) *Delegated Healthcare Activities and the Commissioning of Adult Social Care*. https://www.skillsforcare.org.uk/resources/documents/Developing-your-workforce/Care-topics/Delegated-healthcare-interventions/Delegated-healthcare-activities-and-the-commissioning-of-adult-social-care.pdf (accessed August 16, 2024).

Tingle, J., and McHale, J. (2007) *Law and Nursing*. London: Elsevier.

Communicating with patients

5

Communication is a huge topic, and there are many very good books available on the subject.

The purpose of this chapter is to raise awareness of the issues around communicating with patients and consider some of the ways by which we can improve our skills to enable us to become more *effective* communicators, and thereby improve our patient care.

WHY IS GOOD COMMUNICATION SUCH AN INTEGRAL PART OF EFFECTIVE HEALTHCARE?

There is plenty of evidence for the potential benefits of effective communication in healthcare. Although most of the following references are a little old now they still hold true. When the patient understands what is going on, and feels that they have been listened to and that they have some element of control over their fate, there are many potential benefits, including the following.

- Improved compliance (now usually referred to as concordance) with treatment and improved clinical outcomes (Beach et al. 2006).
- Higher levels of patient satisfaction with fewer complaints (Clever et al. 2008).
- Better information-gathering from the patient.
- Reduction in pain and anxiety (Dougherty and Lister 2015).
- Reduction in unnecessary or inadequate treatment, and subsequent reduction in cost. (McDonald 2020).
- Higher levels of job satisfaction for the healthcare worker (McGilton et al. 2006).

What is communication?

I have struggled to find a definition of communication that says or communicates exactly what I feel is important. There are many definitions

DOI: 10.4324/9781003460381-8

available for the term in general and some more specific definitions for what it means in the realms of healthcare. Life itself depends on people communicating effectively with each other, whether it is verbal or non-verbal, and all healthcare must have good communication at its core. When we are with other people, we are constantly communicating either by talking, using the tone and volume of our voice, as well as the actual words, or through our body language, gestures and facial expressions. We can also communicate a message or an impression through our choice of clothes and general appearance (see Box 5.1).

Box 5.1 Methods of communication

Verbal and written

- Talking face-to-face or on the phone
- Tone/volume of voice
- Sign language
- Lip-reading
- Text, email, letter, fax
- Books, media, information leaflets

Non-verbal

- Active listening – hearing what is being said or not being said
- Touching
- Body language, gestures, facial expressions
- Appearance, dress
- Music

Problems may occur when the meaning of the message is lost or mis-understood, or maybe never received in the first place.

We all like to think of ourselves as good communicators but may be surprised to discover how often patients take the wrong message away with them. So, what are we doing wrong?

The actual *understanding* that takes place is perhaps the single most important factor in communication, so the effectiveness of the communication can be measured by the similarity behind the idea transmitted and the message that has been received. In other words, has the receiver (i.e., the other person or group of people) understood and taken away the message we want to convey?

It is often said that the single biggest problem in communication is the illusion that it has taken place – and I think we can all second that!

Verbal communication

When we talk to patients, there are several factors to take into consideration. We must make sure that the following describes what we say.

Appropriate to the age and level of understanding of the patient.

Accurate: Only ever give advice or information from objective and evidence-based resources. When you don't know something or are unsure about the accuracy of your information, refer the patient to the appropriate health professional.

Clear: Make sure that what you say is unambiguous so that the patient is left in no doubt about your instructions. Always ask the patient if they understand and if they have any questions.

Honest: Avoid false reassurance.

NON-VERBAL COMMUNICATION

How we say something is just as important, if not more so, than *what* we say. We must be aware of the potential effect non-verbal communication may have on our patients. It has been suggested that 93% of 'emotional meaning' is found in a person's facial expressions and tone of voice, and only 7% is from what a person says (Borg 2010).

Following are some points to think about.

- *Be aware of your facial expressions*: Even a subtle movement in the facial muscles, such as a raised eyebrow, can imply surprise or criticism, and may make the patient feel uncomfortable because they may feel as if they are being judged.
- *Think about body posture*: If you fold your arms and cross your legs, this is called closed body posture, and will not encourage a patient to open up and talk, but if you adopt an open body posture or mirror the way your patient is sitting (see Figure 5.1), they will feel more comfortable and talk more freely. Try it out on your friends and see what happens! Of course, there may be times when closed body posture is necessary: if, for example, a patient is very chatty and you need to get on with your work.
- *Watch your gestures*: Pointing a finger can come across as very aggressive or patronising. There are some cultural differences to be aware of, too. 'Thumbs up' is not necessarily a friendly gesture, and in Greece, for example, it may be considered quite rude.

Essential Knowledge and Skills for Healthcare Assistants

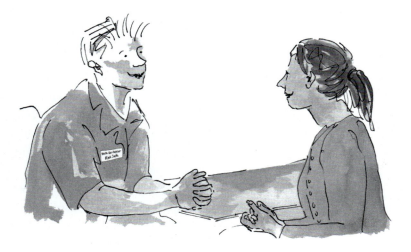

Figure 5.1 HCA with patient

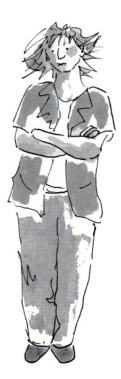

Figure 5.2 Untidy HCA

- *Consider your appearance*: What are you communicating to your patients if you turn up at work with your hair untidy and with a dirty uniform on? You might have just been in a rush, but the chances are that your patient will conclude that you are uncaring or slapdash in your approach. This is not a good start in a consultation, and may not give your patient much confidence, and it may not actually convey the type of person you are at all (see Figure 5.2).

Are you a good listener?

Have you ever had a conversation with someone who is *not* a good listener? They just seem to be waiting for you to finish so that they can make their own comments, and they are not actually listening to what you are saying. How does this make you feel? Do you enjoy talking to these people?

Really listening, or 'actively listening', to what someone is saying – and sometimes more importantly to what they are *not* saying – is a skill that takes practice. It is often difficult to listen properly when you are busy or distracted, but it is well worth it in terms of what you can learn about your patient. It also makes them feel that you care about them and that they are valued. Maintain eye contact and avoid the temptation to look at the computer or at your watch while the patient is talking. At intervals during the consultation, reflect and summarise back to the patient what you think they have told you to check that your information is accurate and to show that you have been listening, such as the following.

So, Mr Jones, just to clarify, you said you had been feeling unwell for three weeks now and your pain is getting worse?

OVERCOMING BARRIERS TO COMMUNICATION

There are many barriers to effective communication. Sometimes there is nothing we can do about these, but often there are things we can do that will help, such as the following.

- *Consider practical difficulties*: For patients with impaired hearing or sight, physical disabilities or learning difficulties, it might be useful to write or type information clearly or in large type size. Always face the patient, speak clearly and never shout. There are many resources available for patients with various types of disability. There are leaflets in Braille for the blind, leaflets in different languages and for patients who may not be able to read or have a learning disability, and leaflets that include drawings to explain various clinical procedures.
- *Consider fear, pain, anxiety and fatigue*: Remember, many patients feel vulnerable and alone when faced with illness. They may appear to be

aggressive or may be unable to take in much information if they are frightened or in pain. Be tolerant and understanding, and avoid giving more information than necessary until the patient is calm or feels better. It is our role to try to reduce the patient's anxiety and build their confidence when we can.

- *Avoid interruptions and distractions*: Turn the phone to silent and make sure the room is private and free from distraction. Discourage colleagues or patients from knocking on the door when you are with a patient.

- *Avoid medical terminology*: Talk in a language your patient can understand. Working in the clinical environment, we become very used to medical jargon and forget that to our patients it is sometimes like a foreign language. Avoid medical terms and always check that your patient understands what you are talking about.

- *Check for mismatched agendas*: Is your agenda the same as your patient's? For example, you may want them to stop smoking, but they may not have any intention of stopping. They may want to discuss their depression when your remit is to record their blood pressure. Try to make sure you are both there for the same purpose or effective communication becomes difficult (see Box 5.2).

- *Consider possible personality clashes*: Do some patients get on your nerves or rub you up the wrong way? Never mind how hard we try, there will always be some patients we cannot get on with and some that make our heart sink. Keep your attitude professional and calm. Avoid confrontation and check that the pitch of your voice doesn't rise, indicating irritation. Try some of the assertiveness techniques discussed in Chapter 6. Alternatively, if there is someone you really cannot get on with, you may need to make sure this patient is booked in with someone else if possible.

- *Consider language and cultural differences*: If the goal of providing safe, high-quality care is to be achieved, you must address linguistic and cultural barriers to communication with patients. Your own culture affects your understanding of a word or sentence and even your perception of the world. This can seriously interfere with the effectiveness of the communication process with people from different cultures (Schyve 2007). There can be misunderstanding and lack of respect for people whose cultural values are different. As a care provider, you owe it to your patients to be aware of your own cultural values and biases, and to be alert to the misunderstandings that may occur as a result. If the patient does not speak English, you may need to utilise an appropriate resource for interpretation, such as LanguageLine (2024).

- *Avoid overfamiliarity*: You may feel you are just being friendly or trying to relax a patient by using an endearment such as 'my love' or 'darling', or by using their first name instead of giving them their full title. However, this sort of language may be interpreted by the patient as overfamiliar or disrespectful. My mother is a good example here. She is 95 and really hates anyone using endearments instead of her name when she goes for her hospital appointments. Other patients may not have a problem with it, but always ask permission before calling a patient by their first name and avoid the use of endearments. Take care not to invade a patient's body space or touch them inappropriately. While you may be very tactile in your personal relationships, you should keep a distance in professional relationships. To use my mother as an example again, one consultant she sees always puts his arm around her and he sometimes hugs her. He also always comments on how marvellous she is for her age. No doubt he thinks he is being pleasant and putting Mum at ease when in fact it is having the opposite effect and she finds it very embarrassing and now dreads seeing him. Touching someone gently on the arm can be useful to show that you care, but more than this is rarely appropriate.

In summary, communication should be patient-centred and responsive to the patient's needs, preferences, beliefs and values. To communicate effectively with patients, we should endeavour to:

- choose the best method to communicate;
- remove the barriers to communication when possible;
- stop to ask questions, clarify and check understanding;
- listen sincerely and with empathy and warmth;
- consider cultural differences; and
- know our audience and respect them.

Box 5.2 Case study: a breakdown in communication

Jenny the HCA was helping the nurse run the diabetic clinic. She performed the physiological measurements before the patient saw the nurse. She would often be in the same room when the nurse was talking to her patients, and realised it made her feel quite uncomfortable. On one occasion, the nurse was telling the patient off. She spoke quite loudly and sounded like a teacher addressing a naughty child, rebuking him for indulging in a high-fat diet. The man sat back, folded his arms and crossed his legs. He was polite but said little throughout the consultation. At the end of the appointment, when the patient had left, the nurse sighed and said, 'How can we help these patients when they won't help themselves? I feel like I'm banging my head against a brick wall most of the time'.

Jenny privately sympathised with the patient, and she wondered how much – if anything – he had learnt or benefited from the appointment.

In this situation, the nurse had created a barrier to effective communication by patronising the patient instead of engaging him as an equal partner in the consultation. It would have been helpful to explore why he chose to eat unhealthily and assess his readiness for change. If he indicated an awareness of his unhealthy diet and a willingness to change, she could then have provided him with the appropriate written information. By adopting an authoritative stance and treating him as if he was stupid, she alienated her patient and he clearly demonstrated disengagement by his closed body language. The message the nurse intended to send was not received and communication broke down.

WHAT ABOUT PATIENTS WITH DEMENTIA?

Dementia is a term that is used to describe a collection of symptoms that include problems with communication, as well as memory loss, problems with perception and reasoning, and problems coping with everyday activities. It is a huge problem all over the world, and the size of the problem is constantly increasing. In the UK alone, it is estimated that the incidence of dementia currently stands at around 944,000 people, and this is expected to rise to over a million by 2030 because people are living longer; around 1 in 11 people age 65 and older have dementia (NHS 2023a).

My father had Alzheimer's (which is one type of dementia), and I saw first-hand how this illness can devastate not only the person who has it, but also the family, the carer and everyone involved. My father was a proud, kind and very intelligent man, and to see him reduced to a frightened and aggressive shadow of himself was a truly awful experience. I saw as well how ill it made my mother, who succeeded in caring for him at home against all the odds until the last two weeks of his life. It was so worrying when we finally had to concede defeat and have him admitted to a care home. We needed to know that the staff there understood what a lovely man there was underneath the man they saw, who was ravaged by his disease. We needed to know that they would preserve his dignity and speak to him as an intelligent man. I wrote a poem to try to make the staff in the home aware of my dad's various problems and foibles, and to make them aware of the person beneath the old man with dementia, which is unfortunately all they would see and know of him.

My poem for Dad when he was admitted to a nursing home with dementia:

PLEASE LOOK AFTER ME

My name is John and here's my rhyme,
I hope you'll spend a little time
To get to know me and my ways
And learn about my bygone days
To start with, please bear this in mind
I don't eat meat of any kind.
But you'll be glad – I do eat fish
I love my food, I'll scrape the dish!
Now my right ear is very sore
So, if you touch it I might roar.
My feet are very tender too
Take care or I might swear at you.
My right hand hurts – arthritic pain
Be gentle please or I'll complain.
If I lash out I hope you'll see –
It's just my illness, it's not me,
For under all the hurt and pain
I'm frightened and my addled brain –
No longer functions as it should,
Believe me I so wish it would.
I'm husband, dad, granddad as well
Much loved by all, hope you can tell.
Remember I was once like you
With life before me, laughter too
I really was a clever man
I had a business, had a plan.
I'd play the piano, paint and dance
Played bowls and golf and took the chance –
To water-ski and ski on snow
Did lots of things, so now you know
I'm not the man I used to be
I now need help, please care for me.

27/7/13, Zoë (John's daughter – who thinks the world of her dad)

Communicating with a person with dementia

Considering how common the problem of dementia is now, you will almost certainly come across a patient with this disease at some stage in your career. Because of this, you really need to try to work out how to care for and communicate with these patients. The best way to learn about this is to look out for and attend any workshops or training you can access on dementia. Understanding what it involves and how it affects the patient is a larger topic than I have room for in this book, but it will really help you when you communicate with these patients in the future.

There are many useful resources with tips about how to communicate with patients who have dementia. Two that I have found particularly useful are the Alzheimer's Society (2024) and the NHS (2023b). They have produced some guidelines that may help you when communicating with the patient with dementia, and I've summarised them for you in what follows.

Some useful tips

- To begin with, you need to *relax and slow down*! You'll be thinking a lot faster than the person with dementia, and will put them under pressure without realising if you're not careful.
- *Introduce yourself.* They may not know you, even if you know them well.
- *Stay positive, respectful and friendly*, and *never* patronise them or ridicule them. Be careful about correcting mistakes or getting impatient. It is usually easier to answer the same question repeatedly rather than point out that you've already told them the answer many times. It is also easier to agree with them rather than cause them stress by correcting them, but if necessary you can try offering an alternative if they get something wrong. For example, if the patient thinks it might be winter when it is the middle of August, you might offer an option for them such as, 'Do you think it might be summer now as the sun is shining and it's quite warm?'. Remember, though, that confrontation is usually pointless and will only lead to frustration for both parties.
- *Speak slowly and clearly, using short sentences.* Give simple choices and give them time to respond.
- *Be patient* and calm, and try not to interrupt. Give them your full attention and make sure that you maintain eye contact as far as possible during the conversation.
- *Use the person's name as much as possible*, as this will help remind them that you are talking to them.

Communicating with patients

- *Encourage them to join in conversations with others* when possible and let them speak for themselves, especially during discussions about their welfare or health.
- *Acknowledge what they have said*, even if they don't answer your question appropriately – show that you've heard them and encourage them to say more. Try rephrasing questions if they don't understand the first time.
- *Keep an appropriate distance to avoid intimidating them*, but you might also feel it appropriate to touch or hold their hand to reassure them (you must make an individual judgement here to work out what feels right for that patient).
- *Be more aware of non-verbal messages* such as facial expressions and body language. Is there any indication that they are in physical discomfort or pain, or distressed in some other way?
- *Minimise distractions* as far as possible, because people with dementia often find it more difficult to concentrate when there is background noise.
- *Have pictures or objects in front of you that will help*. For example, if discussing medication, have it there with you or have a picture of it.
- *Try to put yourself in their position* and work out how they might be feeling, and don't shy away from tears. Stay with the person and offer support. Say how you think they feel (e.g. 'You look sad right now').
- *Remember that the patient with dementia can find it very difficult to find the right words.* So, if they say 'I need my mum', it might be that they are feeling scared and unattached rather than specifically referring to their long-dead mother.
- When you finish the conversation, *shake their hand* and let them know that you've enjoyed your time together and the conversation you had.

And remember, you might be that person with dementia one day. How would *you* like to be treated?

Footnote

I now find myself caring for my husband who has been diagnosed with Alzheimer's, and although I like to think I might be better equipped to deal with it now, it is still a challenge and different in many ways to the experience I had with my father. This may be due to the difference in their personalities and in our relationships, but it highlights for me that while guidance on communicating with dementia patients is very helpful for healthcare workers, it remains a constant personal learning curve for the carer – and it's worth remembering that no two people with dementia are the same.

REFERENCES

Alzheimer's Society (2024) *How to Communicate with a Person with Dementia.* https://www.alzheimers.org.uk/about-dementia/symptoms-and-diagnosis/symptoms/how-to-communicate-dementia#content-start (accessed August 16, 2024).

Beach, M., Keruly, J., and Moore, R. (2006). Is the quality of the patient provider relationship associated with better adherence and health outcomes for patients with HIV? *Journal of General Internal Medicine* 21(6): 661–665. https://pubmed.ncbi.nlm.nih.gov/16808754 (accessed November 7, 2024).

Borg, J. (2010) *Body Language: 7 Easy Lessons to Master the Silent Language.* London: FT Press.

Clever, S., Jin, L., Levinson, W., and Meltzer, D. (2008) Does doctor–patient communication affect patient satisfaction with hospital care? Results of an analysis with a novel instrumental variable. *Health Services Research* 43(5 Pt 1): 1505–1519. http://www.ncbi.nlm.nih.gov/pmc/articles/PMC2653895/ (accessed August 16, 2024).

Dougherty, L., and Lister, S. (2015) *The Royal Marsden Manual of Clinical Nursing Procedures* (9th ed). Oxford: Wiley-Blackwell.

LanguageLine (2024). https://www.languageline.com/uk (accessed August 16, 2024).

McDonald, A. (2020) *Improving Communication Between Healthcare Professionals and Patients in the NHS England. Summary Report.* https://www.england.nhs.uk/wp-content/uploads/2021/07/SQW-NHS-Improving-Communication-Summary-Report.pdf (accessed August 16, 2024).

McGilton, K., Irwin-Robinson, H., Boscart, V., and Spanjevic, L. (2006) Communication enhancement: Nurse and patient satisfaction outcomes in a complex continuing care facility. *Journal of Advanced Nursing* 54(1): 35–44.

NHS (2023a) *What is Dementia?* https://www.nhs.uk/conditions/dementia/about-dementia/what-is-dementia (accessed August 16, 2024).

NHS (2023b) *Communicating with Someone with Dementia.* https://www.nhs.uk/conditions/dementia/living-with-dementia/communication (accessed August 29, 2024).

Schyve, P. (2007) Language differences as a barrier to quality and safety in health care: The joint commission perspective. *Journal of General Internal Medicine* 22(Suppl. 2): 360–361. https://www.ncbi.nlm.nih.gov/pmc/articles/PMC2078554 (accessed August 16, 2024).

Simple assertiveness skills

Many HCAs find themselves in a difficult position when they have previously been working as a receptionist or on the administrative team in the same place of work. They are used to doing work for the doctor or nurse, often without questioning, based on the supposition that in clinical matters, the nurse or doctor knows best. In their new role, they must be able to refuse to accept a task if they feel as if it is outside their sphere of competence. Some doctors and nurses may not always have a clear idea of what HCAs can and cannot do, and may not understand why the HCA might appear reticent to agree to a new task that may seem very simple and straightforward to them. It can also be very flattering when the doctor or nurse have such faith in their HCA and assume that they will be more than happy and capable to take on a new role. The HCA might then feel as if they are in some way letting down their medical colleagues or disappointing them if they are doubtful about their own ability and refuse to accept a delegated task. They may also find themselves in the same position with reception staff or patients who now see them in a clinical domain, and so view them as 'a nurse' and therefore assume them capable of advising on complex health issues. The HCA must develop the ability to say no assertively when necessary, without appearing awkward or lazy and without creating confrontation or confusion.

WHAT IS ASSERTIVENESS?

Let's think about what assertiveness is. Maybe you have heard the term directed at somebody who comes across as a bit bossy or overconfident. It is a term that is often misused and is even used as a term of abuse at times. This is because it is being confused with aggressiveness, but in fact it is quite different, and it is essential to understand that difference (see Figure 6.1).

If you are *assertive*, this means that you're acting in your own best interests but also respecting the rights and feelings of others. You should be able to express positive and negative feelings comfortably without

DOI: 10.4324/9781003460381-9

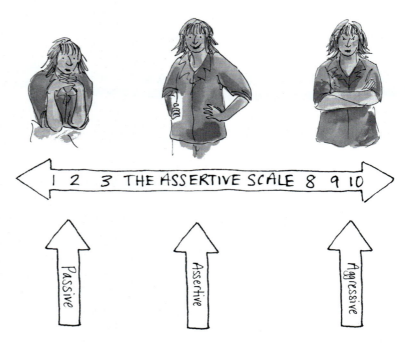

Figure 6.1 Assertiveness scale

undue anxiety. *Aggression*, by contrast, usually involves an attempt to dominate others, with the aggressor standing up for their own interests at the expense of the rights of others. Aggression ignores or dismisses the needs, wants and opinions of others. It can take many forms, including verbal abuse, physical abuse, manipulation, bullying, emotional blackmail, exclusion of others and judgemental attitudes, to name but a few. So the main difference between assertiveness and aggression comes down to how the words or behaviour affects the rights and well-being of the person on the receiving end.

The other end of the spectrum is when we act *passively*. In this case, we are failing to stand up for our rights or doing so ineffectively. We might express our needs or opinions in an apologetic, self-effacing way. We will try to avoid conflict and try to please others. This type of behaviour may be more of a problem for the HCA who is new to the role and anxious to please.

In either case, whether we behave aggressively or passively, the results can be equally harmful to ourselves and those we are interacting with.

To be truly assertive, we must:

- decide what we want;
- decide if it is fair;
- ask clearly for it;

- not be afraid of taking risks;
- be calm and relaxed;
- express our feelings openly;
- give and take compliments easily; and
- give and take fair criticism.

(Lindenfield 2001)

Saying no

Perhaps the most important thing to learn first is how to say no. So, when a colleague or patient asks you to do something that you feel inadequately prepared for, try the following.

- Notice your gut reaction. If you are in doubt, then say so without giving excuses. If you feel unsure, then ask for more time to consider the request, but if this latter response is just playing for time when you know your answer should have been no, then don't prevaricate. Say so directly and calmly, without raising your voice (see Figure 6.2).
- If saying no puts the requester in a difficult position, think of possible alternatives that you are trained to do that may help. For example, if a doctor asks you to do an injection when you are not competent to do so, refuse politely, but offer to fetch the injection for the doctor to do it or offer to make another appointment for the patient to come back for the nurse to do it.

Broken record technique (Smith 1975)

This is an old but still very useful technique in many different situations, such as responding to cold-callers or sales people, returning faulty goods, and refusing to take on an inappropriate task.

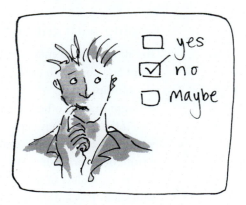

Figure 6.2 Assertiveness: saying no

For example, if a patient asks you to break confidentiality, how will you say no?

Mrs Brown: While I'm here, can you tell me the results of my husband's blood tests, please?

Susan: I'm not able to give you any information without Mr Brown's consent.

Mrs Brown: But that's ridiculous – we're married and don't keep any secrets from each other. Please give them to me.

Susan: There are very clear rules on confidentiality, and I cannot break them, so I'm not able to give you that information without Mr Brown's consent.

Mrs Brown: This is quite outrageous – I think I'll have to report you to the practice manager unless you give me the results.

Susan: I am sorry if you're upset about this Mrs Brown, but I cannot give you that information without Mr Brown's consent. If you would like to speak to the practice manager about it, then perhaps we can come to some other arrangement with your husband's consent, so that we can give you his results in the future.

The same phrase, maybe with slight alterations or explanation, is repeated in a calm, relaxed manner. Take care to start with the mildest stance, only becoming more assertive if necessary. Avoid jumping in with an aggressive or passive stance. If you need time to think the request over, then say so. If you practise this technique on the next cold-caller, you will be amazed at how quickly they give up! But as with all assertiveness techniques, you need to practise.

Coping with criticism

One more assertiveness tip that is worth developing is the ability to accept and cope with criticism. This can help you in personal and work relationships.

Accept that the other person has the right to criticise you. Now determine if the criticism is fair and hopefully constructive or unfair in which case it may be delivered condescendingly or be designed to belittle you in front of others. If it is fair and valid criticism, then accept it and learn from it, regardless of how it may have been made. Separate the content (which may be valid) from the way it is given, and don't take it personally.

If it is unclear, then challenge it calmly and rationally and ask for clarification: 'I'd like you to give me some examples of what you mean'.

Most importantly, if it is invalid or unfair, then don't take it on board. Never beat yourself up and allow your self-esteem to be battered by unfair or invalid criticism. You might choose to respond by using an 'I' statement (e.g. 'As I see it . . . ') or you might choose to ignore it. But however you respond, do not allow it to affect you.

There is not enough space in this one chapter to go through all the different ways of developing and improving your assertiveness skills, but I hope this has given you some food for thought. Remember your rights and responsibilities, and keep calm!

There are lots of very good resources online that are worth exploring for more information on how to be assertive, and there is a wealth of books on the subject. Start with a few small changes and build on those. Remember, you also have the right to be non-assertive when it suits you – providing this doesn't violate anybody else's rights, of course!

ACTIVITY

Now read the following passage and try to answer the questions.

Penny has just taken on the role of HCA, having previously worked on reception. She is doing a busy blood clinic and notices that she has too many patients squeezed in so that she struggles to get her clinic finished on time for the samples to be collected. Later that day, the laboratory technician rings the surgery complaining that the samples have been incorrectly labelled. Over the course of the next month, the same thing keeps happening, but Penny does not like confrontation and is reluctant to complain about the situation. She puts her head down and soldiers on, and hopes that everyone will notice how hard she works without complaining. She feels terrible because she is constantly rushing and cannot do her job properly. She blames the girls on reception, who she feels must be jealous of her new role and are trying to make life difficult for her.

The laboratory staff have complained three times about incorrect labelling, and because of this, the practice manager asks Penny to explain herself. He criticises her for not pointing out how busy she was and not attempting to rectify the situation. Now she feels even worse and as if the whole world is against her.

How is Penny behaving?

How could she have acted assertively to change this situation?

Suggested answers to the activity are presented in Box 6.1.

51

Box 6.1 Suggested answers to activity

> Penny is acting in a passive way in the mistaken belief that people will be pleased with her efforts to cope with the workload. Instead of this, she makes mistakes and people around her become irritated and annoyed with the mistakes she is making. She is also compromising patient care. As a result, she feels unhappy and undervalued.
>
> ## Acting assertively
>
> - Arrange a meeting with the practice manager.
> - Print off the overbooked clinic lists as evidence of the problem.
> - Identify how many of the bloods were urgent and how many could have been booked in a later clinic.
> - Calmly point out that it is not possible to practise safely under this sort of pressure.
> - State calmly and clearly the time required to perform and label a blood test safely.
> - Make an action plan together to address this problem.
> - Document the outcome of your meeting.
> - Evaluate the outcome after a specified time.

REFERENCES

Lindenfield, G. (2001) *Simple Steps to Getting What You Want*. London: Thorsons.

Smith, M.J. (1975) *When I Say No, I Feel Guilty: How to Cope Using the Skills of Systematic Assertive Therapy*. Bantam USA.

Confidentiality, consent and record-keeping

Working in a healthcare setting with members of the public is a very responsible role, and you must be aware of your legal obligations and your patients' rights. The three most important issues pertaining to the legal aspects of your role are confidentiality, consent and record-keeping. This chapter will unpick each of these concepts, and will provide a few useful tips to enable you to fulfil your legal obligations and to ultimately protect your patient and yourself. Legislation relevant to the topics to be discussed is listed in Box 7.1.

Box 7.1 Current legislation

- Data Protection Act (2018)
- The Caldicott Principles (National Data Guardian for Health and Social Care 2020)
- Equality Act (2010)
- NHS Code of Practice. Confidentiality (Department of Health 2023)
- Freedom of Information Act (2000)
- Computer Misuse Act (1990)/Computer Misuse (Amendment) Act (2022)
- Mental Capacity Act (2005)/Mental Capacity (Amendment) Act (2019)
- Access to Health Records Act 1990 (Revised 2023)

CONFIDENTIALITY

As a healthcare assistant, you will already have some understanding of the importance of confidentiality and of the potential repercussions for you and the patient when confidentiality is broken. Anyone with access to patient information must have a contract that clearly stipulates the principles of confidentiality and the resulting disciplinary action that could result when those principles are not adhered to. This chapter will consider how to maintain confidentiality when dealing with patient information.

DOI: 10.4324/9781003460381-10

What is confidentiality and why is it so important?

Confidentiality is a fundamental part of professional practice.

It is the legal obligation that is derived from statutory and case law, as well as forming part of the duty of care to a patient (Beech 2007).

Patients have a legal right to expect that any information they give to a healthcare professional will be used only for the purpose for which it was given and will not be disclosed to others without permission. It is important because the patient is in a vulnerable position and is dependent on the healthcare worker. There must be trust in this relationship if the patient is to offer vital information and comply with treatment.

There is a great deal of legislation that has been developed to protect this right (see Box 7.1).

Disclosure

Disclosure means the giving of information, and requires consent from the individual if it is to be lawful and ethical. If possible, consent should be freely and fully given by the information-giver. The only exception here is where there is a statutory obligation to disclose or if that disclosure can be justified as being in the public interest (GMC 2024).

This may be, for example, when there is a risk of significant harm to individuals or groups, or society in general (e.g. child abuse, drug trafficking or other serious crime).

Sometimes information may be shared with other people or organisations not directly involved in the person's care on a 'need to know' basis. In this case, the patient must be aware that this information is to be shared, unless the health worker feels there may be a violent response (see Box 7.2).

In some cases, information may be withheld from a patient if the clinician considers that it would cause serious harm to the physical or mental health of the patient or would breach the confidentiality of another patient.

Box 7.2 Case study: disclosure

> Susan, the healthcare assistant, was seeing Jenny, a patient who was three months pregnant. Jenny had attended for a blood test, but while there she confided that she was taking amphetamines. Susan was very concerned about the potential risk to the baby

and advised the patient against taking such drugs. She documented the consultation carefully but did not explain to the patient that this information would now be available to other healthcare professionals. When consulting the doctor a week later, Jenny happened to see her notes on a poorly positioned computer screen and was very upset to see what had been written. She complained that this information was confidential and she had not thought it would be documented. In this case, the HCA was right to document the information because of the potential risk to the unborn child, but she should have made it clear to Jenny that she would have to disclose this information to other health professionals. She should also have spoken to the person in the surgery responsible for safeguarding (see Chapter 8).

The Caldicott Report

The Caldicott Report on the Review of Patient-Identifiable Information (Department of Health DoH 1997) was commissioned by the Chief Medical Officer when there was concern regarding the increasing use of information technology resulting in the easy dissemination of patient information. The report principles have now been increased to eight and are as follows.

- Justify the purpose for collecting the information.
- Use patient-identifiable information only when necessary.
- Use the minimum necessary confidential information
- Access to patient-identifiable information should be on a strict 'need to know' basis.
- All health workers who have access to patient information should be aware of their responsibilities.
- Comply with the law.
- The duty to share information can be as important as the duty to protect patient confidentiality
- Inform patients and service users about how their confidential information is used.

(National Data Guardian for Health and Social Care 2020)

It is now a requirement for every NHS organisation to have a Caldicott Guardian. These are members of staff with the responsibility for ensuring the Caldicott principles are adhered to and all patient data is kept secure.

Avoiding accidental breaches of confidentiality

You may not mean to breach confidentiality, but when you're busy and distracted, it is all too easy to do so without realising. Observing a few simple rules will help guard against this.

Never leave records (including those on the computer screen) unattended where they may be read by unauthorised persons. Clear your desk at the end of the day and turn off your computer or put it into password-protected mode.

Never discuss matters relating to patients outside of the clinical setting or discuss a case with a colleague in public when it may be overheard or seen by others from outside the clinical setting, such as on social networking sites. Remember that anything you write on social networking sites is never private and can never be completely deleted. There have been well-documented cases of nurses who have made this mistake and lost their jobs as a result. Healthcare workers should never put confidential patient information online or post inappropriate comments about patients, and the Nursing and Midwifery Council (NMC) have produced a leaflet on social media guidance for nurses which is worth a read (NMC 2023).

Watch out for accidental breaches of confidentiality. For example, take care when talking to friends outside of work not to disclose the fact that you saw a mutual acquaintance in the surgery.

Think about telephone confidentiality. Avoid talking to patients on the phone in areas where personal information can be overheard by other patients (see Figure 7.1).

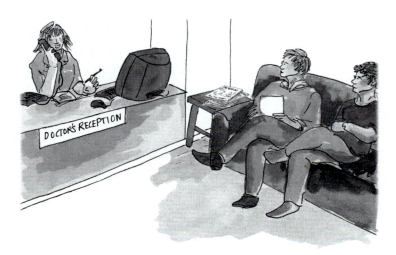

Figure 7.1 HCA not observing confidentiality

Always gain the patient's consent before you leave messages on an answering machine or with other family members. It can be helpful to use code words to make sure you are talking to a specific person and not just someone who is claiming to be that person.

Remember, if information is passed to another party without consent, the patient may be able to bring a civil claim for breach of confidentiality against the health worker's employer and demand compensation.

CONSENT

Before any examination and before providing any treatment or care, you must obtain consent. You can never assume a patient has given you informed consent just because they are sitting in front of you and appear to be implying that they consent. Do they *understand* what the procedure involves, why it is being done, and what the possible benefits, risks and alternatives are? Do they understand the consequences of not receiving the proposed treatment? If they don't understand the information, then they cannot give informed consent. If anything goes wrong following the procedure, you run the risk of being charged with battery (a form of assault), or you may be accused of negligence.

The whole process of establishing consent must be rigorous and transparent (see Box 7.3).

Box 7.3 Case study: consent

Carole the HCA was good at taking blood, but on one occasion the patient developed a large bruise following the procedure. He complained to the practice manager and threatened to seek compensation from the practice for injury. It was discussed as a critical incident, but there was no suggestion that Carole's technique was to blame in this instance. It was understood that bruising is always a potential complication following venepuncture, and may be due to inappropriate activity too soon afterwards as much as to problems during the procedure or poor technique. To avoid any problems in the future, it was decided that patients would be given a short information leaflet outlining possible risks, including possible bruising, and the aftercare required following the procedure to reduce this risk. This would ensure that the patient had the necessary information available to be able to give informed consent, with an understanding of what was being done and the possible risks. It was also an opportunity to provide written information about the required aftercare to the venepuncture site,

> advising against heavy lifting or excessive movement within four hours.
>
> This could have resulted in a claim against the surgery because failure to warn of risk is considered as negligence. There is quite a high chance of bruising in this case, but the harm is usually minimal. From a legal point of view, such a claim would be unlikely to succeed as it is very likely that if told of the risk, the patient would have consented to having the blood test done anyway. Nevertheless, it has the potential to create a great deal of stress and anxiety for all involved.

Capacity is the term used to denote the patient's ability to use and understand information and to decide on whether they want to proceed, and then to communicate that decision.

We assume that every adult has the capacity to give informed consent unless the following apply.

- They are unable to take in or retain the information.
- They are unable to understand the information.
- They are unable to use the information to decide on whether to proceed.

When giving information about a procedure, it must be given in a way that is understandable to that patient. They must have enough time to consider this information and be given the opportunity to ask questions if they want to. We should regard the patient as a partner in the caregiving process and uphold their right to make decisions about the type of care and treatment they receive. We must also respect their decision to decline treatment even if we feel that this is not in their best interest. If your patient declines treatment, always refer them back to the nurse or doctor, as they may need more detailed information to enable them to decide what course of action to take.

Consent must be given freely, and never under duress or under influence from the health professional or family or friends. It can be withdrawn at any time during the procedure, in which case the procedure must be stopped immediately.

Make sure that you accurately document discussions that relate to obtaining consent.

Types of consent

Verbal consent is usually sufficient for tasks that will be performed by the HCA working at level 3.

Written consent is needed when the procedure is lengthy, risky or complex. This provides evidence of the fact that discussions have taken place and of the patient's decision, but it does not necessarily protect the clinician. If the patient can subsequently prove that they did not have an adequate explanation or they were coerced or rushed into signing the consent form, the consent may be considered invalid.

Who cannot give consent?

Children younger than the age of 16

Legally, a person is not considered an adult until they are aged 18 or older. However, people between the ages of 16 and 18 can consent to or refuse medical treatment.

In England and Wales, children younger than the age of 16 cannot consent to or refuse treatment, as they are considered to lack the capacity, and only the person with parental responsibility can give or refuse consent on their behalf. Sometimes, if the child is considered to have significant understanding and intelligence so that they can make an informed decision about their treatment, this rule may be overturned. For contraception and sexual health issues, there is a set of guidelines called the Gillick Competency and Fraser Guidelines (NSPCC 2022) that clearly set out the criteria required for children under the age of 16 to be able to consent to their own treatment without the involvement of their parent(s).

In Scotland, the parent's consent cannot override the refusal of a child younger than 16 to treatment when the medical practitioner considers that the child can understand the nature and potential consequences of the treatment.

I have had many discussions with HCAs regarding whether it is appropriate for them to be performing procedures such as venepuncture or ear irrigation on children under the age of 16. Although this is not specifically related to consent, it is perhaps a good time to mention it. There are no hard and fast rules about this, and it will depend on your local protocol and on whether the child will cooperate. Whenever you are in any doubt, always refer to the nurse or doctor.

Who can give consent for children under 16?

In recent years, HCAs have started to assist with the administration of intranasal influenza vaccines to children aged from 2 years up, and if you are one of those who has received the appropriate training and will be performing this task, it is very important that you understand who can give consent for the child to have this.

Consent for younger children can be given by the person who has *parental responsibility* (if that person has capacity and is able to communicate their decision). When that person brings the child in response to an invitation for immunisation and presents that child for immunisation, then this is normally considered as evidence of consent. They will usually have had a discussion with the health visitor and/or GP previously and will have signed a consent form.

The mother will normally have parental responsibility, but the father will only have parental responsibility if he was married to the mother when the child was born, or if he subsequently marries her or he is named as the father on the child's birth certificate. Parental responsibility can also be granted to the father by the court, or there may be a Parental Responsibility Agreement signed by both parents witnessed by an officer of the court.

Immunisation should only be carried out if both parents agree or if there is a specific court approval that the immunisation is in the best interests of the child.

The person with parental responsibility does not need to be present. The child may be brought by someone else such as a grandparent or childminder, but take care in this case and make sure consent has been obtained previously from the person with parental responsibility. If unsure, then you should contact them to confirm their consent.

When you are in any doubt, always refer to the registered nurse for advice.

People who are mentally incapacitated

Never make assumptions that a person is unable to make decisions or give informed consent based on their diagnosis, appearance or behaviour. When there is any doubt, the medical practitioner in charge of that person's care should make the decision based on the person's best interests.

No one else can give consent for a person, although the medical practitioner will usually involve close relatives to try to determine what the wishes of the person may have been if they previously had capacity, for example when the person has dementia. Sometimes the patient may have made advance decisions on how they wish to be treated if they suffer loss of capacity. They may also choose to appoint another person to make these decisions for them, which involves completing a legal form called the 'Health Care Power of Attorney'.

The Mental Capacity Act (2005) outlines the assessment required to determine if a person is mentally capable of decision-making, and the Mental Health Act (2007) describes the rare circumstances when a patient can be hospitalised or treated against their wishes.

In summary

- Always gain consent before carrying out any care or procedure on a patient.
- Make sure that the consent is valid. The patient must have the capacity to consent and you should clearly explain the procedure in a way that the patient can understand, including what is being done, why it is being done, and the potential risks and benefits.
- Refer the patient back to the doctor or nurse if the patient refuses or withdraws consent.
- Seek advice if you are unsure about the consent for a child.
- Document that you obtained consent.

RECORD-KEEPING

Good documentation is an integral part of care. There is a legal requirement to 'do and document', and the law places an equal value on both. Too often, we consider documentation to be a chore and afford it a lower priority compared with the actual task, but instead we should use it as a tool to transmit and receive information, and thereby ensure good-quality safe care for our patients. Good record-keeping has many important functions. It promotes:

- high standards of care and improved continuity of care;
- better communication and dissemination of information within the team;
- an accurate account of treatment, care planning and delivery;
- the ability to detect problems or changes at an early stage;
- clinical audit, research and allocation of resources; and
- the ability to properly address any complaints or legal processes.

Remember, the quality of your record-keeping reflects the standard of care you give, and good record-keeping usually indicates a safe and skilled practitioner. Remember as well that whatever you write in a patient's notes becomes a public record, so take care with your documentation (see Figure 7.2).

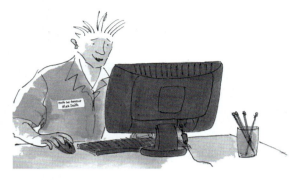

Figure 7.2 HCA at a computer

Good record-keeping: the process

You should record:

- what you saw or observed beforehand;
- the process explained to the patient, including potential risks and benefits;
- informed consent obtained;
- what you did;
- what you saw afterwards; and
- the advice that you gave.

Record-keeping should adhere to the following principles.

- Documentation should be legible and signed if handwritten. If digital, it must be traceable to the person who provided the care that is being documented (e.g. by using their personal login).
- Registered nurses will be delegating the task of record-keeping, and may countersign entries made by trainee HCAs or APs (until that HCA/AP is deemed competent in record-keeping), but only if they have witnessed the activity.
- Record the event as soon as possible and at least within 24 hours.
- Time and date the record as close to the actual time as possible.
- Keep it simple, relevant and accurate. It should be clear and unambiguous, without jargon, speculation or assumptions. Never make subjective statements about a patient.
- Only use abbreviations if they are accepted and understood by everyone.
- Involve the patient in the documentation process when possible so that they are aware of what has been written.

> When you record an event, think of the record being scrutinised in a court of law. If this ever happens, it probably won't be until a year or two after the event happened, so it will be difficult for you to remember details of the event. And remember, if it isn't documented, then in the eyes of the law, it never happened!

- Record any problems that occurred and the action that was taken to deal with them.
- Never delete or amend records without a full and signed explanation of why this was done.

(RCN 2023)

ACTIVITY

Look back on your record-keeping for your last few patients. Be constructively critical and try to decide what was good or bad about the various entries.

- Was your meaning clear? Did you include all the relevant information?
- Was there any unnecessary waffle or jargon?
- Did you use any abbreviations? If you did, would they be understood by everybody?
- Did you make any subjective comments about your patient?
- Did you include that you obtained consent (assuming that you did, of course)?
- Do you need to make any changes to your documentation for the future?

REFERENCES

Access to Health Records Act 1990 (Revised 2023). https://www.legislation.gov.uk/ukpga/1990/23 (accessed September 2, 2024).

Beech, M. (2007) Confidentiality in health care: Conflicting legal and ethical issues. *Nursing Standard* 21(21): 42–46. https://pubmed.ncbi.nlm.nih.gov/17305035 (accessed November 7, 2024).

Computer Misuse Act (1990). https://www.legislation.gov.uk/ukpga/1990/18/contents (accessed August 29, 2024).

Computer Misuse (Amendment) Act (2022). https://www.dataguidance.com/sites/default/files/computer_misuse_amendment_act_2022_assent.pdf (accessed August 29, 2024).

Data Protection Act (2018). https://www.legislation.gov.uk/ukpga/2018/12/contents/enacted (accessed August 16, 2024).

Department of Health [DoH] (1997) *The Caldicott Committee Report on the Review of Patient Identifiable Information*. https://webarchive.nationalarchives.gov.uk/ukgwa/20130124064947/http:/www.dh.gov.uk/prod_consum_dh/groups/dh_digitalassets/@dh/@en/documents/digitalasset/dh_4068404.pdf (accessed September 2, 2024).

Department of Health (2023) *Confidentiality Code of Practice*. https://assets.publishing.service.gov.uk/media/5a7c13f0ed915d210ade16fb/Confidentiality_-_NHS_Code_of_Practice.pdf (accessed November 23, 2024).

Equality Act (2010). https://www.legislation.gov.uk/ukpga/2010/15/contents (accessed August 23, 2024).

Freedom of Information Act (2000). https://www.legislation.gov.uk/ukpga/2000/36/contents (accessed August 29, 2024).

GMC (2024). *Disclosing Patients' Personal Information: A Framework.* https://www.gmc-uk.org/professional-standards/professional-standards-for-doctors/confidentiality/disclosing-patients-personal-information-a-framework (accessed September 2, 2024).

Mental Capacity Act (2005). https://www.legislation.gov.uk/ukpga/2005/9/contents (accessed August 29, 2024).

Mental Capacity (Amendment Act) (2019) *Liberty Protection Safeguards LPS.* https://www.gov.uk/government/collections/mental-capacity-amendment-act-2019-liberty-protection-safeguards-lps (accessed August 29, 2024).

Mental Health Act (2007). https://www.legislation.gov.uk/ukpga/2007/12/contents (accessed September 2, 2024).

National Data Guardian for Health and Social Care (2020) *The Eight Caldicott Principles.* https://assets.publishing.service.gov.uk/media/5fcf9b92d3bf7f5d0bb8bb13/Eight_Caldicott_Principles_08.12.20.pdf (accessed August 23, 2024).

NMC (2023) *Social Media Guidance.* https://www.nmc.org.uk/standards/guidance/social-media-guidance (accessed September 2, 2024).

NSPCC (2022) *Gillick Competency and Fraser Guidelines.* https://learning.nspcc.org.uk/child-protection-system/gillick-competence-fraser-guidelines (accessed September 2, 2024).

RCN (2023) *Record Keeping: The Facts.* https://www.rcn.org.uk/Professional-Development/publications/rcn-record-keeping-uk-pub-011–016 (accessed September 2, 2024).

Safeguarding

8

There is an increasing awareness of the importance of safeguarding in all walks of life, and this is especially true in your role as an HCA where you will meet many vulnerable patients who may be at risk of harm from others. Safeguarding adults and children is integral to your duty of care. You must be able to recognise the signs and symptoms of abuse in your patients and to report on them appropriately.

In this chapter, I'll unpick some of the safeguarding theory, using information from RCGP (2019), RCN (2019, 2024) and CPD (2024), and try to offer some clear guidance as to how you can identify when there may be a safeguarding issue and what you then need to do about it. However please remember this is an overview. It simply isn't possible to include all the information you need in this chapter, so you must attend all the safeguarding training provided by your local health authority.

WHAT DOES SAFEGUARDING MEAN?

Safeguarding is essentially about protecting people from harm or abuse. Such abuse may include any of the following: physical, psychological/emotional, sexual, financial or material abuse, neglect, self-neglect, honour-based violence, female genital mutilation (FGM), discriminatory abuse, organisational abuse and modern slavery.

As an HCA, it is highly likely that at some time you will encounter someone who is at risk or suffering from abuse or neglect which may be deliberate or could be the result of ignorance or lack of training.

A BRIEF HISTORY OF SAFEGUARDING

In 2003, Ian Huntley was convicted of the murder of two school girls in Soham, Cambridge. He had been employed as caretaker of a college where he had regular contact with children despite having a criminal record which included nine sexual offences. An independent inquiry chaired by Sir Michael Bichard was subsequently set up to identify how

DOI: 10.4324/9781003460381-11

Huntley came to be employed and how such a tragedy could be avoided in the future (The Bichard Inquiry Report 2004). As a result of this report, the Vetting and Barring Scheme was developed to protect children and vulnerable adults ('Adults at risk') by preventing people who may pose a risk of harm from working or volunteering with them. The report recommended that all people working with vulnerable groups should be registered, requiring a vetting procedure to filter out people who are deemed unsuitable. The scope of this vetting and barring procedure was extended by the Safeguarding Vulnerable Groups Act (SVGA) in 2006.

The Deprivation of Liberty Safeguards (2009) provided an amendment to The Mental Capacity Act of 2005 with a legal framework to protect those who lack capacity to consent to certain aspects of their care (see Chapter 7).

Safeguarding in healthcare was affected by the Care Act (2014), which describes the statutory responsibility requiring integration of care and support between health providers and local authorities. It also lists the six key principles of safeguarding, as follows.

- Accountability – if you are ever entrusted with information which you think might indicate that some sort of abuse is occurring, you should inform the individual that you will have to report your concerns. The Data Protection Act of 2018 does not prevent you from sharing information about a child or vulnerable adult if you consider them to be at risk of harm.
- Empowerment – for the abused person so that they feel they have control over their situation. Your support and encouragement are important to achieve this.
- Partnership – via your Practice Manager and Lead GP with the Local Authority or whoever can help you with detecting and reporting abuse.
- Prevention – when you can detect potential abuse and report something in time to prevent it from happening or getting worse.
- Proportionality – when you understand how to report your concerns appropriately according to the level of risk presented.
- Protection – you may need to act as ally or advocate for patients who have experienced abuse or who may be at risk of it. If you can support them and represent their interests appropriately, you may be able to protect them from further harm.

There are now designated professionals with specific roles and responsibilities for safeguarding children and part of their role is to provide strategic advice and guidance to the various health boards and services.

WHO MIGHT BE AT RISK?

There are number of factors that can increase the person's vulnerability to abuse including things such as very young or very old age, disabilities or health problems (mental or physical), frailty, substance misuse or chronic stress (parent or carer), domestic abuse, lack of engagement with services, previous abuse or neglect, history of abuse or of offending (parental or carer) and being in the care of the Local Authority (i.e. a 'looked after child'). Adults who are physically dependant on others or who have a sensory impairment or a learning disability, those who have low self-esteem, drug or alcohol problems or those who have bad experiences of disclosing abuse are also vulnerable to abuse.

Anyone can abuse or neglect including partners, family members, carers, acquaintances, paid staff, volunteers, strangers, children and people who exploit adults seen as vulnerable.

WHAT IS THE ROLE OF THE HCA?

As an HCA, you should be able to demonstrate an appropriate level of competence for safeguarding of adults and children. As a minimum, you should be able to know which groups of people are likely to be at risk and the signs or symptoms that may indicate possible harm. You also need to know who to seek advice from if you have any concerns.

You must attend regular safeguarding training at least every two years and take part in continuing professional development (CPD). Your manager should review your safeguarding knowledge annually and organise refresher courses if needed.

Your role is the following.

Recognise abuse – spot the signs

There are many possible signs and symptoms of abuse, including the following.

Physical signs such as bruises in unusual areas, bite marks and slap marks. These may not tie up with the history as given by the carer or parent or the abused person. Other physical signs may include inappropriate dress, dirty or unkempt appearance, signs of poor nutritional health, signs of deliberate self-harm or drug use.

Physical sexual signs that may include soreness in genital and anal areas, sexually transmitted infections or an underage pregnancy. Female genital mutilation (FGM) may present as difficulty walking, sitting or standing and reluctance to undergo normal medical examinations.

Bullying, especially when there is a power imbalance and when there is repeated behaviour with a deliberate intention to hurt or humiliate and which has a detrimental physical or emotional effect on the victim.

Other signs can include parents or carers not seeking or delaying medical treatment when the vulnerable child or person is ill or injured. There may also be conversational clues such as the person or child talking about being left alone or with inappropriate carers or strangers, or they may express concern for younger siblings without explaining why.

In organisations, there may be danger to workers when health and safety rules have been broken or when there is a lack of resources or products.

Respond to and report suspected abuse

Even if your concern seems minor, it is still important to report it, because early intervention can sometimes prevent a problem from escalating. Whenever you feel there may be a problem, from something you've seen, heard or been told, you should report it via your local safeguarding procedure. You must have a reasonable belief that abuse is current, historical or might happen sometime in the future.

If you think someone may be at risk of imminent harm, you must report your concerns immediately.

The NHS has Safeguarding Leads for Adults and Children and your GP practice or place of work will have a named doctor or nurse to take the professional lead on safeguarding. These people will have had special training to deal with any concerns around safeguarding. They should take your concerns seriously and will either report the issue for you or support you in reporting it. You should be kept up to date with any required action and the outcomes.

Different Health Boards and Trusts will have different methods of reporting, some with online forms and some with paper forms (multi-agency referral forms), but they will all be submitted to the Local Authority where the incident occurred. If queries occur out of hours and there is no suitable person available, Health Board or Trust staff should be able to contact the Local Authority directly via the Out of Hours Team.

Record it

Always keep an accurate record of your concerns and the action that you took.

Safeguarding

Refer

If the risk is urgent and somebody may be at harm immediately, you must refer the patient. In this instance, and if there is nobody available for you to report it to, you should contact the relevant Local Authority or the police.

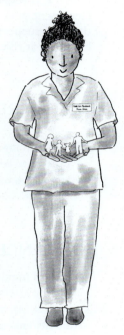

Figure 8.1 HCA safeguarding

Box 8.1 HCA safeguarding

> An elderly couple, Jim and Mary, present for flu/COVID-19 injections. You've met them before, but this year, Mary has changed. She was always quite chatty and cheerful, but on this occasion, even when you try and talk to her, she appears very withdrawn and slightly confused. Jim appears embarrassed by his wife's behaviour. He always seemed to be the dominant partner, but this time he is very overbearing and bullying in his behaviour. When Mary is a little slow removing her coat, Jim shouts at her, roughly removes Mary's coat and apologises to the HCA for his wife being so old and stupid. You're very concerned because Mary says very little and you find yourself worrying about her.
>
> In this instance, Mary is at risk from psychological abuse because of Jim's bullying and aggressive manner, and she is possibly at risk of physical abuse, as well. She is elderly and appears to be suffering with

69

> dementia and she is therefore vulnerable. Jim may be behaving this way because he is tired or not receiving any help to look after Mary, but he is clearly not coping well with the situation. His bullying and rough behaviour and Mary's withdrawn behaviour are clear symptoms of abuse – and this is therefore a safeguarding issue. You should report it as soon as possible to the safeguarding lead in your practice. Document your concerns and the action you took. Hopefully with the right support in place, Jim will be able to cope and Mary will no longer be at risk.

TIME TO REFLECT

Using a Framework for Reflection (see Chapter 2), try reflecting on a situation when you or a colleague reported suspected abuse. What was the outcome, and what did you learn?

REFERENCES

The Bichard Inquiry Report (2004). https://dera.ioe.ac.uk/id/eprint/6394/1/report.pdf (accessed August 2, 2024).

Care Act (2014). https://www.legislation.gov.uk/ukpga/2014/23/contents/enacted (accessed September 7, 2024).

CPD (2024) *Safeguarding Guide for GPs*. https://cpdonline.co.uk/safeguarding-guides/safeguarding-guide-for-gps/ (accessed August 2, 2024).

Data Protection Act (2018). https://www.legislation.gov.uk/ukpga/2018/12/contents/enacted (accessed August 16, 2024).

Deprivation of Liberty Safeguards DoLS (2009). https://www.mentalhealthlaw.co.uk/Deprivation_of_Liberty_Safeguards (accessed August 2, 2024).

Mental Capacity Act (2005). https://www.legislation.gov.uk/ukpga/2005/9/contents (accessed August 29, 2024).

RCGP (2019) *Good Practice Safeguarding in General Practice*. https://www.rcgp.org.uk/blog/good-practice-safeguarding-in-general-practice (accessed August 2, 2024).

RCN (2019) *Safeguarding Children and Young People: Roles and Competencies for Healthcare Staff*. https://www.rcn.org.uk/professional-development/publications/pub-007366 (accessed October 24, 2024).

RCN (2024) *Adult Safeguarding: Roles and Competencies for Healthcare Staff*. https://www.rcn.org.uk/Professional-Development/publications/rcn-adult-safeguarding-roles-and-competencies-for-health-care-staff-011–256 (accessed October 24, 2024).

Safeguarding Vulnerable Groups Act (2006). https://www.legislation.gov.uk/ukpga/2006/47/contents (accessed August 2, 2024).

Health promotion
The key messages

As a healthcare assistant, you are increasingly at the front line of care and in constant contact with patients from all walks of life who are either healthy or unhealthy, or somewhere in between, depending on your and their points of view.

This chapter will offer some guidance on current messages for healthy living that are evidence-based and applicable to most of the adult population. Patients requiring more in-depth health promotion for complex problems should be referred to the nurse, doctor or other health worker with training in health promotion.

WHAT IS 'HEALTH'?

Health is a very subjective thing and hard to define. One of the most quoted definitions of health is from the World Health Organization (WHO 1948), describing it as being 'a state of complete physical, mental and social well-being and not merely the absence of disease or infirmity'. This is still the definition as used by WHO – despite criticism about the use of the word 'complete', which is widely considered as unachievable for most people in the world and which implies that people with any sort of illness cannot be considered 'healthy'. A newer – and I feel more acceptable – definition of 'health' has been suggested as 'the dynamic balance of physical, mental, social and existential well-being in adapting to conditions of life and the environment' (Krahn et al. 2021).

Health promotion has also been defined in several different ways. WHO (2024) define *health promotion* as: 'The process of enabling people to increase control over and to improve their health. It moves beyond a focus on individual behaviour towards a wide range of social and environmental intervention'. NICE (2024) defines health promotion as: 'Giving people the information or resources they need to improve their health. It can also involve changing the social and environmental conditions and systems that affect health'.

DOI: 10.4324/9781003460381-12

As a healthcare assistant, you are well placed to offer healthy living advice to patients, to enable them to move towards that state of 'optimal health' (if that is what *they* want), but you must make sure that the advice is objective and based on current evidence. Use leaflets from objective sources, such as NICE guidelines, the British Heart Foundation, Patient. info and so on. Avoid using leaflets that are endorsed by companies with products to sell, such as some cholesterol-lowering products. By giving out such leaflets, you are inadvertently condoning the consumption of such products. When you are wearing a uniform and a badge that says 'Healthcare Assistant', patients will assume you know what you are talking about. Avoid the temptation to offer them advice if you don't have very good evidence to back up your information.

When offering health advice, you should also consider where the patient is on the cycle of change, as originally developed by Prochaska and Di Clemente (1992). It is an old model with some limitations, but still widely used today, and most people involved in promoting health are very familiar with it (see Figure 9.1).

If the patient is in the pre-contemplative stage, then 'brief intervention advice' is recommended, raising awareness and offering help if required for the future. This is in accordance with the NICE guidance, which advises on the need to recognise when people may be more open to change, such as when recovering from a behaviour-related condition

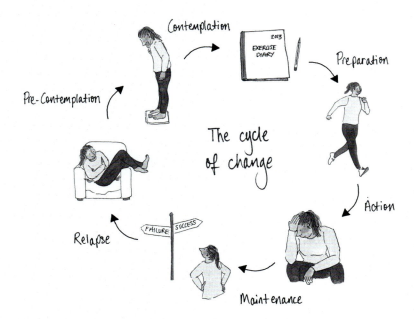

Figure 9.1 Cycle of change

or when becoming a parent (NICE 2014). Conversely, the health worker must also recognise when offering behavioural change may not be appropriate due to personal circumstances. NICE (2014) recommends that primary care workers use brief interventions for health promotion advice to motivate people to change behaviours that may damage their health. For example, if the patient smokes, ask them how interested they are in quitting. If they want to stop, refer them to an evidence-based smoking cessation service.

Even 'brief intervention advice' requires a degree of skill and training in health promotion techniques, and you should take care not to step out of your area of skill and competence.

As health professionals, it is our role to offer advice when a patient wants or needs it. But even when *we* feel as if they need our advice, they still have the right to refuse it. We should aim to empower our patients by giving them the information, but remember their right to live their lives the way they choose.

If the patient is moving into the contemplation stage or is preparing to change, this is when they are most likely to be receptive to healthy living messages.

WHAT'S GOING ON IN THE WORLD OF HEALTH PROMOTION?

There is a lot going on, and there are many resources and guidelines available to help you in this complex area of healthcare. Some examples of recent innovations include the following.

- Public Health England (PHE) in 2016 adopted an approach to behaviour change called 'Making Every Contact Count' (MECC), which was developed in the East Midlands in 2014. It is based on the premise that organisations and individuals have millions of daily interactions with other people, and can utilise these opportunities to support those people in making positive changes to their physical and mental health and well-being. The idea is that small actions with lots of people will result in big population changes. It is still considered to be a useful form of health promotion, and there are plenty of online learning resources (PHE 2016).
- NHS England (2024a) provide e-learning for healthcare and a 'Toolkit for MECC', which are available online.
- NHS England (2024b) provides free e-learning that covers brief interventions for alcohol and tobacco use.

- Public Health England (PHE 2023) has produced a resource for healthcare professionals who are working with patients to prevent illness, protect health and promote well-being. The resource provides tips on having brief conversations, health coaching and motivational interviewing.

These resources are evolving and are constantly updated. Make use of them! Key areas for promoting health include:

- healthy eating and alcohol awareness;
- increasing activity levels; and
- smoking cessation.

HEALTHY EATING AND ALCOHOL AWARENESS

There are many well-documented benefits of healthy eating (see Box 9.1). The *Eatwell Guide* (NHS 2022) has now replaced the *Eat Well Plate*.

The latest guide simplifies the healthy eating message and demonstrates a well-balanced diet with the emphasis on 'good' foods. Foods higher in fat, salt and sugar – such as crisps, biscuits, cakes and sweets – appear at the end of the guidelines with the advice that they are not needed in the diet and should be eaten in only very small amounts.

Box 9.1 Benefits of healthy eating

- Lower cholesterol.
- Weight control.
- Good bowel function.
- More energy.
- Reduced risk of some chronic disease (e.g. heart disease, diabetes).
- Stronger teeth and bones.
- Lower blood pressure.
- Clearer skin.
- Improved immunity.

TIPS FOR HEALTHY EATING

This advice is suitable for most people, but may vary for groups of people with specific health problems, pregnant women or those with special dietary requirements. They should be referred to the dietician or some-one with specialist knowledge if necessary.

The information in the following tips has been adapted from the *Healthy Eating* advice leaflet produced by Patient.info (Hudson 2023).

Some tips for healthy eating include the following.

1 **Cut down on trans fats and saturated fats.** For many years, we have blamed fat for the obesity epidemic and other health problems because fat contains about twice as many calories as carbohydrate or protein per gram. However, we now know that the picture is more complex than this, and it seems likely that carbohydrates play a larger role in weight gain than previously realised. Even so, it is probably still a good idea to eat less fat when trying to lose weight. The main source of the trans fats is in processed foods, when hydrogen is added to vegetable oils to make them more solid, and they occur in foods such as hard margarines, biscuits, pastries and cakes, fried foods and processed foods. They can increase the 'bad' low-density lipoprotein (LDL) cholesterol, which is associated with heart disease and diabetes. Saturated fat is found in meat and should be replaced with unsaturated fats such as in oily fish, avocado and olive oil. Choose fats labelled as monounsaturated or polyunsaturated, such as olive oil or sunflower oil. Avoid frying food, choose lean cuts of meat and watch out for hidden fats in foods such as pastries, cakes and biscuits.

2 **Eat at least two portions of fruit and three portions of vegetables per day.** The Patient.info advice leaflet on losing weight suggests 7–9 portions of a variety of fruit and vegetables in place of foods that are higher in fat and calories (McKechnie 2023a), with some authors suggesting a corresponding reduction in the risk of strokes, heart disease and some cancers (Aune et al. 2017).

3 **Eat at least two portions of oily fish per week.** Oily fish contains Omega-3, which is important for a healthy heart, blood vessels, lungs and immune and hormonal systems (BDA 2024). Other sources of Omega-3 include walnuts, pumpkin, flax and chia seeds, soya milk, soya beans and tofu.

4 **Eat whole grains and nuts regularly.** Eating whole grains as part of a low fat diet appears to substantially reduce the risk of heart disease, stroke, Type 2 diabetes and bowel cancer. The increased fibre from whole grains also helps you feel fuller for longer and reduces snacking which may help to maintain a healthy body weight. (BDA 2022) Nuts also provide a source of healthy fats, protein, minerals, vitamins and fibre.

5 **Limit salt intake to less than 6g per day.** Action on Salt (2023) discusses the 'overwhelming evidence' pointing to the importance of

salt reduction on improved health, whereby salt reduction can save thousands of deaths from heart disease and strokes.

6 **Limit alcohol to less than 14 units per week.** Alcohol in excess can lead to a variety of problems (see Box 9.2). As alcohol has become more readily available in supermarkets, with prices much lower compared with those in pubs or restaurants, more people are choosing to drink alcohol at home on a regular basis. This has led to an increase in alcohol-related disease and addiction. Alcohol also contains calories so choose healthier non-alcoholic drinks and keep within recommended limits spread evenly over several days with at least two alcohol free days a week. For information on units and tips on how to cut down on alcohol, check out the leaflet 'Alcohol and Sensible Drinking' (McKechnie 2023a).

7 **Avoid processed meats, 'ready meals' and ultra-processed food (UPF).** This includes things such as crisps, mass produced packaged bread, margarines and spreads which contain added chemicals such as emulsifiers and preservatives. Basically if a product contains more than five ingredients not typically used in home cooking, it is probably best avoided. Current evidence, although not yet conclusive, suggests that these foods may be bad for us (BHF 2024a).

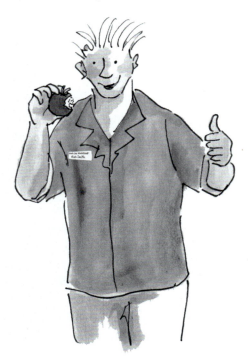

Figure 9.2 HCA eating an apple

8 **Avoid sugar-sweetened drinks, sweets and cakes** (all of which are high calorie but nutritionally poor). Try not to add sugar to tea, coffee and cereals. Use fruit as an alternative to add sweetness to recipes. Give children water or milk as their main drink. Keep chocolate or sweets for an occasional treat. This is in line with mounting evidence, especially regarding added sugar in the diet, clearly pointing to an increased risk of obesity in adults and children (Cohut 2018), diabetes, heart disease and dental caries. Added sugar has also been associated with some cancers, possibly through the link with obesity (Huang et al. 2023).

The debate about protein

We know that protein is important in the diet for energy, growth and repair of cells, but it is now recognised that we generally eat a lot more than we need – and while this isn't necessarily a problem, it depends where it comes from. Diets heavy in meat have been linked to heart disease, diabetes and some cancers (BHF 2024b).

It is recommended that dietary protein comes from a variety of sources, especially the lower-fat options such as chicken, fish, lean meat, tofu, beans, pulses and soya.

And what about carbohydrates?

Until fairly recently, we were advised to base our meals on starchy carbohydrates such as potatoes, pasta, rice or bread, but this advice is changing because we now know that some carbohydrates (especially those that are processed) can have adverse effects on blood sugar, insulin levels and weight. The patient.info leaflet suggests that about a third of our diet should be made up of complex starchy carbohydrates, preferably high fibre options such as whole meal bread, whole grain cereals and brown rice (Hudson 2023). These foods have a lower glycaemic index which means that they are processed by the body in a way that is less likely to cause obesity or diabetes.

HOW DO WE HELP OUR PATIENTS LOSE WEIGHT?

It seems as if the normalisation of 'plus-size' body shapes may be leading to an increasing number of people underestimating their weight, which is undermining the efforts to tackle the problem of obesity in England and presumably elsewhere (Muttarak 2018). First, you need to establish if your patient needs to lose weight (and persuade them of this!), and if so, how much they need to lose. Measure their height, weight and waist (see Chapter 12). It is also useful to work out the basal **metabolic rate** for each patient to determine how many calories they need. Although government guidelines suggest that men can have 2,500 calories and women 2,000 calories each day, this is a generalisation and cannot be applied to everyone. Obviously, people who have active jobs will need more calories than those in sedentary work.

When your patient says that they have tried everything but nothing works, this probably isn't true. Any diet that involves eating fewer calories *will* work if it is maintained, so the secret is finding the 'diet', or better still finding the change in eating habits, that can be enjoyable and maintained. Nobody will stick to eating just cabbage for very long! Some top tips for helping your patients to lose weight are included in Box 9.3. These are taken from an information leaflet provided by the British Obesity Society. These are worth checking out as a useful resource for your patients. They are very readable and straightforward, with humorous and colourful diagrams, and they are available in different formats depending on the gender and ethnicity of your patient. (Copies of the leaflet can be obtained from: info@britishobesitysociety.org.)

Another useful patient.info leaflet with tips for how to achieve weight loss is available online (McKechnie 2023b).

Don't forget that in the end, it is your patient's responsibility to lose weight and not yours! Check where they are on the cycle of change (see Figure 9.1). Sometimes, I think we take too much on ourselves. I have certainly been guilty in the past of bringing patients back weekly for months on end to try to encourage them to lose weight. If they are not doing their part and losing some weight, this is not a cost-effective use of your valuable time. Be brave and stop following up these patients until they are really prepared to stick to their side of the agreement and reduce their food intake.

Box 9.2 Problems related to alcohol

- Liver disease.
- Stomach ulcers.
- Obesity.
- Malnutrition.
- Dependence.
- Antisocial behaviour, aggression and violence.
- Accidents.

Health promotion

ACTIVITY How closely do *you* adhere to the principles of healthy eating? Try keeping a food diary for a week and write down everything you eat and drink. Be honest! Now compare your eating habits with the guidelines given in this chapter. Is there room for improvement? How will you make changes to improve your diet?

Box 9.3 Top tips for losing weight for your patients

- Weigh yourself – it is easy to convince yourself you're not getting bigger, but scales never lie!
- Think about joining a slimming club such as Slimming World. They are a great way to get support for men and women.
- Find out your body mass index (BMI), and if it tells you that you're obese, then don't try to convince yourself it's muscle – unless it really is!
- Remember, you don't have to diet – just make a few sensible changes.
- Become more aware of how many calories you are consuming. Watch portion sizes.
- Track what you eat – a food diary is helpful, or you could try taking pictures with your phone of every bit of food you put in your mouth throughout the day. There are also many different apps available for this now, and these can make the process of tracking what you eat easy and fun. You will probably be surprised!
- Get competitive with your friends and get fitter to lose weight.
- Avoid fizzy drinks and stick to water instead. Moderate your alcohol intake.
- Eat smaller portions and try to stop eating when you are full.
- Avoid processed foods.
- Try to sit down when you're eating and avoid eating when watching the TV or working.
- Get the whole family involved in cooking.

Adapted from information in the British Obesity Society leaflet available from info@britishobesitysociety.org

INCREASING ACTIVITY LEVELS

Every year, 1 in 6 deaths in the UK occurs as a direct result of physical inactivity, with an estimated cost of £7.4 billion. Physical activity can help prevent and manage more than 20 chronic conditions, including heart disease, some cancers, depression and Type 2 diabetes. Despite this fact, the population of the UK is approximately 20% less active than in the 1960s, and this is set to rise to 35% by 2030 (Office for Health Improvement and Disparities; OHID 2022).

There are many benefits to be gained from exercise and increased levels of activity (see Box 9.4).

PHE produced an evidence-based document outlining an approach to physical activity called *Everybody Active, Every Day* (PHE 2014). This was reviewed in 2021, with some positive progress identified despite problems encountered with limited funding for human and financial resources (PHE 2021).

So what should you be advising your patients regarding how they can become more active? The following information from the NHS guidelines (NHS 2024a) might be helpful. Everyone should engage in moderate or vigorous physical activity every day and should minimise sedentary behaviour, but individual physical and mental capabilities must be considered when interpreting the guidelines.

- *Moderate-intensity activities* include things that will make you breathe harder and increase your heart rate, such as brisk walking or cycling.
- *Vigorous activity* will make you warmer, breathe much harder, and will make your heart beat rapidly, and includes things such as running, swimming, skipping (see Figure 9.3), playing football and climbing stairs. You will not be able to say more than a few words without pausing for breath.
- *Muscle- and bone-strengthening activities* involve working against resistance or using body weight, and include things such as swinging, hopping, skipping, playing tennis, dancing, exercising with weights, carrying heavy loads and chair aerobics.
- *Minimising sedentary behaviour* can be achieved by reducing the amount of time spent sitting down as much as possible. Reduce time spent watching TV, using the computer or playing video games. Take regular breaks away from your desk or couch, and try breaking up sedentary time by swapping long bus or car journeys for walking part of the way.
- *Activities should be enjoyable to the individual*, as they are then more likely to be sustained. Referral to an exercise specialist can lead to longer-term changes in physical activity, and many exercise referral schemes exist around the country based at local leisure centres.

Health promotion

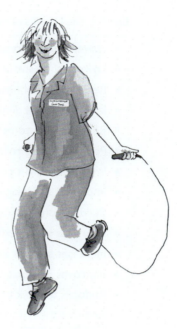

Figure 9.3 HCA skipping

- *Activities to improve balance and coordination* include things such as Tai Chi, Pilates and yoga.
- *For the under-5s*: Physical activity should be encouraged from birth through floor-based and water-based play. Once the child can walk unaided, they should be physically active daily for at least 180 minutes spread throughout the day.
- *For children and young people from 5–18 years*: This age group should be engaging in moderate- to vigorous-intensity physical activity for at least 60 minutes and up to several hours every day. Activities should include muscle- and bone-strengthening activities at least three days a week.
- *For adults*: Over a week, periods of activity should add up to at least 150 minutes of moderate-intensity activity in bouts of ten minutes or more. One way to achieve this would be to do 30 minutes on at least five days a week. Alternatively, 75 minutes of vigorous activity can be spread across the week, or moderate- and vigorous-intensity activity can be combined.
- Include physical activity that will improve muscle strength at least two days a week.
- Older adults should incorporate physical activity to improve balance and coordination at least two days a week.

Box 9.4 The benefits of exercise and increased activity

- Lowers blood pressure.
- Lowers cholesterol.
- Reduces risk of heart disease and Type 2 diabetes.
- Improves bone density.
- Reduces symptoms of depression and anxiety.
- Provides stress relief.
- Improves weight control.
- Improves self-image.
- Builds stronger muscles.
- Improves joint flexibility.
- Increases stamina and energy.
- Improves immunity.
- Reduces the risk of dementia.
- Reduces the risk of breast cancer and colon cancer.

During the writing of this chapter, it occurred to me that I had been sitting at the computer for long periods of time, so I decided to take my own advice and go for a walk. I walked briskly for 30 minutes, and included a steep hill in my walk, so I was warm and puffing slightly by the time I got home. I saw my first primrose of the season and felt my cheeks glow as I walked. I must have had a rush of endorphins because I felt so good (and virtuous!), and I felt re-energised when I sat back down to work. I had also topped up my ultraviolet (UV) light exposure, and thereby improved my synthesis of vitamin D and absorption of calcium as a result. Who could ask for more?

Try to practise what you preach, and you will find it's easier to be more enthusiastic when extolling the virtues of exercise and healthy eating because you know it really works. Patients might be more inclined to take your advice if they can see that you believe in what you say.

SMOKING CESSATION

Some interesting facts and figures:

- About 1 in 8 people in the UK smokes, i.e. 12.9% of the population (Action on Smoking and Health; ASH 2023a), but the good news is that the proportion of the population who smoke has decreased from 45.6% in 1974 (Office for National Statistics; ONS 2022).

Health promotion

- Despite this decrease, smoking remains the single most preventable cause of premature death. About 76,000 people in the UK die each year due to smoking, and about half of all lifelong smokers will die prematurely, losing on average about ten years of life (ASH 2023a).
- The estimated cost to society in England alone is approximately £17.3 billion a year. This includes the cost to the NHS of treating diseases caused by smoking, as well as lost productivity due to premature deaths, smoking breaks and absenteeism (ASH 2023b)
- Smokers spend an average of £2,451 a year on cigarettes (ASH 2023a).
- Smoking is the main contributor to health inequalities in England. The proportion of people who smoked in the most deprived areas of England and Wales in 2021 was more than three times higher than in the least deprived areas (ONS 2023).
- Smoking rates among people with a mental health condition are significantly higher than for the general population, and the association between smoking and mental health becomes stronger relative to the severity of the condition (ASH 2019).
- There are more than 4,000 chemicals in tobacco smoke, many of which are highly toxic, including things such as acetone, arsenic, benzene, cadmium, carbon monoxide, formaldehyde and hydrogen cyanide. It is hardly surprising, then, that smoking is the cause of so much ill health.
- About 4.7 million adults were using e-cigarettes (vapes) in 2023, up from 2.9 million adults in 2017 (ASH 2023c).
- Despite increasing concerns about vapes, they are still being recommended by the NHS as a method of quitting smoking along with standard nicotine replacement therapy as they are not considered to be as harmful as smoking.

Some of the many benefits associated with stopping smoking are listed in Box 9.5.

Box 9.5 The benefits of stopping smoking

- Improved fertility/better chance of having a healthy baby.
- Younger-looking skin.
- Whiter teeth.
- Better breathing.
- Live longer and stay well – stopping smoking reduces the risk of more than 50 different smoking associated illnesses.

> - Less stress.
> - Improved smell and taste, and you smell better.
> - More energy.
> - Healthier loved ones.
> - More money.
> - Ability to travel, work and socialise without worrying about needing a cigarette.
>
> NHS (2024b), ASH (2020)

TIPS FOR ENCOURAGING PEOPLE TO STOP SMOKING

Pre-contemplation (not interested in changing behaviour):

- Accept their position and don't be judgemental.
- Check on their long-term plans: 'Are you planning to continue smoking?'.
- Remind them that support is available if they decide to stop.
- Contemplation (thinking about making a change):
- Encourage the patient to talk about the pros and cons and find their own reasons for quitting.
- Correct any myths, such as 'the damage is done', and remember it is never too late to quit.
- Provide information about local smoking cessation provision.

Preparing to change (ready to change and receptive to advice and information):

- Explain that smoking cessation advisors will support them throughout the process.
- Provide a leaflet on stopping smoking.
- Refer to the doctor for a prescription for nicotine replacement therapy or other medication if appropriate.
- Reinforce the reasons they gave for quitting and give praise and encouragement.
- Refer patients to the local smoking cessation organisation, where these are available.

When I eat too much dessert, I don't post it on Facebook – because if it isn't charted, it didn't happen!

REFERENCES

Action on Salt (2023) *New Research Confirms the UK's Current Salt Reduction Programme is No Longer Fit for Purpose.* https://www.actiononsalt.org.uk/news/news/2023/2023-news-section/new-research-confirms-the-uks-current-salt-reduction-programme-is-no-longer-fit-for-purpose-.html (accessed November 6, 2024).

ASH (2019) *Smoking and Mental Health.* https://ash.org.uk/resources/view/smoking-and-mental-health (accessed September 7, 2024).

ASH (2020) *Stopping Smoking.* https://ash.org.uk/resources/view/stopping-smoking (accessed September 7, 2024).

ASH (2023a) *Smoking Statistics.* https://ash.org.uk/uploads/Smoking-Statistics-Fact-Sheet.pdf (accessed September 6, 2024).

ASH (2023b) *£14 Billion a Year Up in Smoke- Economic Toll of Smoking in England Revealed.* https://ash.org.uk/media-centre/news/press-releases/14bn-a-year-up-in-smoke-economic-toll-of-smoking-in-england-revealed (accessed September 6, 2024).

ASH (2023c) *Use of E-cigarettes (Vapes) Among Adults in Great Britain.* https://ash.org.uk/uploads/Use-of-e-cigarettes-among-adults-in-Great-Britain–2023.pdf (accessed September 7, 2024).

Aune, D., Giovannucci, E., Boffetta, P. et al. (2017) Fruit and vegetable intake and the risk of cardiovascular disease, total cancer and all-cause mortality. *International Journal of Epidemiology* 46(3): 1029–1056. https://pubmed.ncbi.nlm.nih.gov/28338764/ (accessed September 4, 2024).

BDA (2022) *Wholegrains.* https://www.bda.uk.com/resource/wholegrains.html (accessed September 6, 2024).

BDA (2024). *Omega-3.* https://www.bda.uk.com/resource/omega–3.html (accessed September 6, 2024).

British Heart Foundation [BHF] (2024b) *Protein: What You Need to Know.* https://www.bhf.org.uk/informationsupport/heart-matters-magazine/nutrition/protein (accessed September 6, 2024).

British Heart Foundation [BHF] (2024a) *Ultra-Processed Foods: How Bad are They for Your Health?* https://www.bhf.org.uk/informationsupport/heart-matters-magazine/news/behind-the-headlines/ultra-processed-foods (accessed September 6, 2024).

Cohut, M. (2018). *Review Confirms Link Between Sugary Drinks and Obesity.* https://www.medicalnewstoday.com/articles/320493.php (accessed September 6, 2024).

Huang, Y., Chen, Z., Chen, B. et al. (2023) Dietary sugar consumption and health: Umbrella review. *BMJ* 381. https://www.bmj.com/content/381/bmj-2022–071609 (accessed September 6, 2024).

Hudson, R. (2023) *Healthy Eating.* https://patient.info/healthy-living/healthy-eating (accessed September 4, 2024).

Krahn, G., Robinson, A., Murray, A., and Havercamp, S. (2021) It's time to reconsider how we define health: Perspective from disability and chronic condition. *Disability and Health Journal* 14(4). https://www.

sciencedirect.com/science/article/pii/S1936657421000753 (accessed September 2, 2024).

McKechnie, D. (2023a) *Alcohol and Sensible Drinking – Safe Limits of Alcohol.* https://patient.info/healthy-living/alcohol-and-liver-disease/alcohol-and-sensible-drinking (accessed September 6, 2024).

McKechnie, D. (2023b) *Weight Reduction.* https://patient.info/healthy-living/weight-loss-weight-reduction (accessed September 4, 2024).

Muttarak, R. (2018) Normalization of plus size and the danger of unseen overweight and obesity in England. *Obesity* 26(7). https://onlinelibrary.wiley.com/doi/full/10.1002/oby.22204 (accessed September 6, 2024).

NHS (2022) *The Eatwell Guide.* https://www.nhs.uk/live-well/eat-well/food-guidelines-and-food-labels/the-eatwell-guide (accessed September 4, 2024).

NHS (2024a) *Physical Activity Guidelines for Adults Age 19 to 64.* https://www.nhs.uk/live-well/exercise/physical-activity-guidelines-for-adults-aged-19-to-64 (accessed September 6, 2024).

NHS (2024b) *Benefits of Quitting Smoking.* https://www.nhs.uk/better-health/quit-smoking/benefits-of-quitting-smoking (accessed September 7, 2024).

NHS England (2024a) *Making Every Contact Count.* https://www.e-lfh.org.uk/programmes/making-every-contact-count (accessed September 4, 2024).

NHS England (2024b) *Alcohol and Tobacco Brief Interventions Programme.* https://www.e-lfh.org.uk/programmes/alcohol-and-tobacco-brief-interventions/ (accessed September 4, 2024).

NICE (2014) *PH49 Behaviour Change: Individual Approaches.* https://www.nice.org.uk/guidance/PH49 (accessed September 4, 2024).

NICE (2024) *Glossary.* https://www.nice.org.uk/glossary?letter=h (accessed September 4, 2024).

OHID (2022) *Physical Activity: Applying All Our Health.* https://www.gov.uk/government/publications/physical-activity-applying-all-our-health/physical-activity-applying-all-our-health (accessed October 27, 2024).

ONS (2022) *Adult Smoking Habits in the UK: 2022.* https://www.ons.gov.uk/peoplepopulationandcommunity/healthandsocialcare/healthandlifeexpectancies/bulletins/adultsmokinghabitsingreatbritain/2022 (accessed September 6, 2024).

ONS (2023) *Deprivation and the Impact on Smoking Prevalence, England and Wales: 2017 to 2021 Census 2021 Released 2023.* https://www.ons.gov.uk/peoplepopulationandcommunity/healthandsocialcare/druguse alcoholandsmoking/bulletins/deprivationandtheimpactonsmokingpr evalenceenglandandwales/2017to2021 (accessed September 6, 2024).

PHE (2014) *Everybody Active, Every Day.* https://assets.publishing.service.gov.uk/government/uploads/system/uploads/

attachment_data/file/374914/Framework_13.pdf (accessed September 6, 2024).

PHE (2016) *Making Every Contact Count*. https://www.england.nhs.uk/wp-content/uploads/2016/04/making-every-contact-count.pdf (accessed September 4, 2024).

PHE (2021) *Everybody Active, Every Day: 5 Years On*. https://www.gov.uk/government/publications/everybody-active-every-day-5-years-on/everybody-active-every-day-5-years-on (accessed September 6, 2024).

PHE (2023) *All Our Health: Personalised Care and Population Health*. https://www.gov.uk/government/collections/all-our-health-personalised-care-and-population-health (accessed September 4, 2024).

Prochaska, J.O., and Di Clemente, C.C. (1992) Stages of change and the modification of problem behaviours. In M. Hersen, R.M. Eisler, and P.M. Miller (eds), *Progress in behaviour modification*. Sycamore: Sycamore Press.

WHO (2024) *Health Promotion*. https://www.who.int/westernpacific/about/how-we-work/programmes/health-promotion (accessed October 24, 2024).

World Health Organisation WHO (1948) *Preamble to the Constitution of the World Health Organization as Adopted by the International Health Conference, New York, 19–22 June 1946*. https://www.who.int/about/governance/constitution (accessed September 4, 2024).

Keeping it clean

Hand decontamination

10

Many thousands of years ago, a Greek philosopher and physician named Hippocrates laid down the moral code of conduct for medical practitioners called the 'Hippocratic Oath'. Within this oath are the words: 'all patients have the right to receive care and come to no harm'.

As healthcare workers, we all have a responsibility to ensure that we uphold this ideal wherever we work and to keep our patients safe. This chapter will focus on hand hygiene, but remember to think about infection prevention and control in everything you do when dealing with patients. Check your local guidelines for information on dealing with sharps, wearing of personal protective equipment (PPE) and disposal of clinical waste.

SETTING THE SCENE

In the nineteenth century, a Hungarian obstetrician named Semmelweis discovered that the likely cause of infection and subsequent death in his obstetric patients originated from medical students who had performed autopsies, resulting in hand contamination. By contrast, patients cared for by the midwives who had not performed autopsies had much lower rates of infection and death. Semmelweis hypothesised that there must be something on the hands of the medical students that could not be seen, but when passed on to the patient could cause infection. He demonstrated a significant reduction in mortality among his patients when medical students washed their hands in a chlorinated lime solution. Despite this important finding, his medical colleagues would not believe him. He was later committed to a sanatorium, where he died at the age of 47. Twenty years on, Louis Pasteur provided the theoretical explanation, or 'germ theory', of disease.

Now, many years later, we are still guilty of causing infections in patients because of a lack of basic infection control procedures, the most important of which is hand hygiene.

DOI: 10.4324/9781003460381-13

Healthcare-associated infections (HCAIs) are infections that were not present before admission to hospital or contact with healthcare workers in the community. They can affect people of all ages, exacerbate existing or underlying conditions, delay recovery and adversely affect quality of life (NICE 2023).

Approximately 300,000 people acquire an HCAI in England every year (6.4% prevalence) while in Wales the prevalence is 5.5–6% and the cost to the NHS is over £1 billion (Mackley et al. 2018).

Many of these HCAIs are preventable using simple measures, such as:

- good personal hygiene of health staff;
- correct hand decontamination;
- appropriate use of PPE such as gloves and aprons (when necessary);
- correct disposal of sharps;
- correct disposal of clinical waste;
- keeping work areas and surfaces clean and free from clutter;
- isolating patients with specific infections; and
- appropriate use of antibiotics and avoidance of overuse.

All nurses are responsible for ensuring that risks to patients are kept to a minimum and that their care is as safe and effective as possible (NMC 2024), and this obviously applies to all healthcare providers (not just nurses). Everyone has a duty of care to their patients and should observe good infection prevention and control guidelines.

WHAT IS INFECTION?

Infection is caused by microorganisms, usually bacteria, viruses or fungi. These are too small to be seen with the naked eye, but if fully active and present in sufficient quantity and in the appropriate environment, such microorganisms can become **pathogens**, and are then capable of causing infection. All microorganisms can become pathogenic. An example of this is a bacterium called *S. aureus*. This is one of the major causes of HCAI or community-acquired infection (CAI). Approximately 30% of the population may be long-term carriers of this bacterium. It is frequently found in the nose and on the skin, and usually causes no problems. However, if the person (or host) has a cut or abrasion, the bacteria can become pathogenic and cause an infection. It can cause pimples, impetigo or **cellulitis**. If it gets into the bloodstream, it can cause pneumonia, **endocarditis** or severe inflammation of the bones (osteomyelitis).

Similarly, many people may have methicillin-resistant *S. aureus* (MRSA) bacteria on their skin or in their respiratory tract. When they are healthy and their skin is intact, it does not cause a problem. However, if they have an open wound or if their immune system is compromised in some way, the MRSA can become pathogenic and cause an infection that is resistant to many types of antibiotics (Henderson 2016).

S. aureus is a very resilient organism but can be removed by correct hand decontamination.

Many different types of microorganisms live on the skin and hands. Some are referred to as *resident flora* and others are called *transient flora*. Resident flora are microorganisms that tend to stay on the skin. They are more difficult to wash off the hands but are less likely to be harmful. Transient flora are microorganisms that are transferred very easily, and they tend to be more harmful and more likely to cause infection. They can be transferred by touch from person to person or from person to an object that may then harbour the organism. The good news is that these transient flora are also washed off more easily, so a good hand decontamination technique will remove or destroy them.

Infection prevention and control is not about destroying all microorganisms in the healthcare environment, as this is simply not possible. It is about preventing the transfer of those microorganisms that are potentially harmful and that may compromise the patient's safety and well-being.

HOW IS INFECTION SPREAD?

For an infection to occur, the *chain of infection* (see Table 10.1) must be unbroken, and so the aim of infection control is to break the chain. Good hand hygiene, or 'hand decontamination', is the most important way of breaking this chain and preventing the transmission of microorganisms.

If infection is to occur because of indirect contact via the healthcare worker's hands, the organism must have been present on the skin, it must survive on the hands for at least several minutes, hand-washing or antisepsis by the healthcare worker must be inadequate or omitted entirely, and the pathogens on the caregiver's hands must come into contact with another patient, either directly or by being shed into the patient's immediate environment (Teare et al. 2001).

Hand hygiene is the simplest and most important way in which we can reduce the spread of infection, and all healthcare workers – from cleaners through to consultants – have a personal responsibility to undertake adequate hand hygiene.

Table 10.1 The chain of infection

Chain of infection	Example
Source of infection ⇩	• Bacteria • Fungus • Virus
Route of transmission ⇩	Direct contact via bodily fluids, or indirect contact via: • Hands • Equipment • Arthropods (e.g. flies, mosquitos) • Airbourne (e.g. respiratory droplets)
Susceptible host ⇩	• Elderly or very young • Immunosuppressed • Open wound/recent surgery • Chronic disease
Point of entry	• Wound • Mouth/nose/eyes/ears • Vagina/rectum

ACTIVITY

When should you decontaminate your hands?

There are many occasions during a day at work when you should decontaminate your hands. How many can you think of?

Check your answers against those given in Box 10.1.

Box 10.1 Five key moments for hand hygiene

When should you decontaminate your hands? The WHO (2009a) has defined the key moments when healthcare workers should perform hand hygiene. These include:

- before touching a patient;
- before clean/aseptic procedures;

> - after body fluid exposure risk;
> - after touching a patient; and
> - after touching patient surroundings.
>
> You could also have included the following:
>
> - at the beginning and end of each shift;
> - after the removal of gloves;
> - before eating;
> - after going to the toilet;
> - after touching your nose;
> - after handling potentially contaminated linen or equipment; and
> - whenever hands are visibly dirty.

HAND-WASHING: THE PROCEDURE

Remember, nails should be short and clean, with no nail varnish. False nails should not be worn at work. Cover open cuts or lesions with a waterproof dressing, and report any skin conditions that are affecting the hands to your manager for advice.

You can download the National Occupational Standard IPC2 'Perform Hand Hygiene to Prevent the Spread of Infection' to use as a checklist for your competencies (Skills for Health 2022), as follows.

1 Remove wristwatches and bangles and any hand jewellery with ridges or stones that can harbour microorganisms before providing care. When wearing plain rings such as wedding bands, move them when carrying out hand hygiene to reach all microorganisms.
2 Wear short sleeves or roll up sleeves prior to hand hygiene.
3 Use either liquid soap or approved alcohol-based hand-rub products.
4 Hand-washing technique (see Figure 10.1):

   - Wet hands under running water before applying soap.
   - Cover all areas of the hands during washing.
   - Rub hands palm to palm.
   - Right palm over the top of the left hand with fingers interlaced, and vice versa.
   - Palm to palm with fingers interlaced.
   - Rub the backs of the fingers to the opposing palms with fingers interlocked.

Essential Knowledge and Skills for Healthcare Assistants

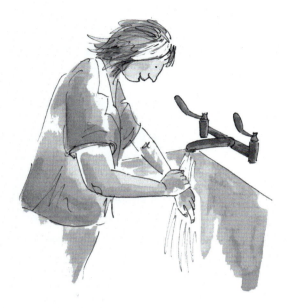

Figure 10.1 HCA washing hands

- Rotational rubbing of left thumb clasped in right palm, and vice versa.
- Rotational rubbing, backwards and forwards with clasped fingers of right hand in left palm, and vice versa.
- Rinse well under running water.
- When lever taps are not available, turn off the tap using a paper towel.
- Dry hands thoroughly using soft disposable paper towels.

5 If your hands are not visibly contaminated with organic matter, it may be appropriate to use alcohol hand-rub. In this instance, follow the manufacturer's guidelines and make sure all areas of your hands are in contact with the gel, using the previously described technique for hand-washing. Allow the gel to dry naturally before contact with the patient.

6 Keep your fingernails short and clean. Do not use nail polish or wear artificial fingernails at work.

7 Before each shift, assess your hands for cuts, cracks and breaks in the skin that could harbour microorganisms.

8 Cover any cuts and abrasions with a waterproof dressing, change the dressing when it appears soiled and keep the area clean to reduce the risk of infection. Never perform wound dressings when you have a cut or abrasion on your hand.

Keeping it clean

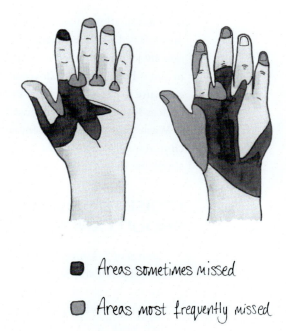

Figure 10.2 Areas missed on washed hands

9   Use hand cream to maintain skin integrity.
10 Report any skin problems to your line manager, occupational health or GP so that you can receive appropriate treatment.
11 Report any difficulties with facilities or supplies for hand hygiene to the appropriate person and ask them to take action to improve the situation.

A video of the correct hand-washing technique is available online (NHS Choices 2021).

Figure 10.2 indicates the most commonly missed areas after hand-washing. Many potentially harmful pathogens could still be present on these hands in the 'missed areas'. Make sure you never miss these areas when you decontaminate your hands.

THE PROBLEM WITH GLOVES

I have a bit of a thing about gloves! I get really annoyed when I see health workers typing on the computer keyboard or answering the phone with their gloves on. I think sometimes people think wearing gloves somehow makes them safer and eliminates the need to decontaminate the hands. Please remember that gloves are no substitute for effective hand decontamination and should only be used *when necessary*. Gloves should only be used when the user is at risk of exposure to blood and body fluids, non-intact skin or mucous membranes where there is the risk of exposure to blood-borne viruses. Gloves should also be worn when there are risks of exposure to chemicals such as cytotoxic drugs and other toxic substances such as NaDCC (commonly used to clean ear irrigation machines).

Wash your hands after removing gloves and discard the gloves in the clinical waste *as soon as the procedure is completed*. All medical gloves are single-use only.

LEGISLATION AND GUIDELINES YOU SHOULD KNOW ABOUT

1 *Control of Substances Hazardous to Health regulations – COSHH 2002* (Health and Safety Executive HSE 2017). Under COSHH, all healthcare workers have a legal duty to assess the risk of infection for employees and patients and all others who may be affected by their work.

2 *Infection Prevention and Control* (NICE 2014). This document provides evidence-based advice on hand decontamination, as well as information on safe management of long-term catheters and vascular access devices.

3 *Surgical Site Infection* (NICE 2019 updated 2020). This document includes information and advice on wound care and the treatment of surgical site infection.

4 *Personal Protective Equipment at Work* (HSE 2022). This document describes the use of PPE for protection of the worker in the workplace.

5 *Guidelines for Hand Hygiene in Health Care* (WHO 2009b). These guidelines are a little old now but are still a useful guide for healthcare workers, administrators and health authorities, with a review of evidence on hand hygiene in healthcare. They make recommendations regarding how to improve practice and reduce the transmission of pathogenic microorganisms to healthcare workers and patients.

6 *Essential Practice for Infection Prevention and Control* (RCN 2017). This document provides evidence-based advice on best practice for prevention and control of HCAIs. It identifies the essential principles for hand decontamination and the use of PPE, as well as the safe use and disposal of sharps and waste disposal.

7 *Aseptic Non-Touch Technique* (ANTT)® (ASAP 2024). This is a framework for aseptic practice that has been developed to improve

the standard of aseptic technique in clinical practice. This is discussed in more detail in Chapter 18.

8 *Find your local trust or health board infection prevention and control policy and read it!* This will include information on things such as hand hygiene, use of PPE, maintaining equipment and the environment, managing blood and body fluid spillages, safe disposal of waste and sharps safety. Your place of work should also have its own policy on infection prevention and control.

TIME TO REFLECT

Try using one of the frameworks for reflection discussed in Chapter 2 to do this.

We know that hand hygiene is the most important measure for reducing HCAIs, but studies on hand hygiene compliance among healthcare workers have repeatedly shown poor compliance with hand hygiene. In NHS England Hospitals, hand hygiene compliance ranges from 40–60% (Over 2023). This is a statistic I find particularly shocking.

1 During your next shift in work, make a note of how many times in the day you decontaminate your hands. If you missed washing or decontaminating after dealing with a patient, why do you think this was?
2 Have a chat with your colleagues and mentor. How many of them decontaminate their hands after every patient encounter or procedure?
3 What would help you and your colleagues adhere to the guidelines more closely?
4 Identify any areas of weakness in your place of work where it is difficult to maintain infection control. Think about things such as not having lever taps, no sink in the treatment area, lack of alcohol hand gel, cluttered work surface, etc. Do any of these apply to your place of work? Or maybe you can think of other problems? Discuss this with the other members of the nursing team and identify an action plan to address these problems.

REFERENCES

Association for Safe Aseptic Practice ASAP (2024). *Aseptic Non-Touch Technique ANTT® Clinical Practice Framework.* https://www.antt.org/antt-practice-framework.html (accessed September 11, 2024).

Health and Safety Executive HSE (2017) *Control of Substances Harmful to Health (COSHH)*. https://www.hse.gov.uk/coshh/index.htm (accessed September 7, 2024).

Health and Safety Executive HSE (2022) *Personal Protective Equipment (PPE) at Work*. https://www.hse.gov.uk/ppe/ppe-regulations–2022.htm (accessed September 7, 2024).

Henderson, R. (2016) *MRSA*. https://patient.info/infections/mrsa-leaflet (accessed September 7, 2024).

Mackley, A., Baker, C., and Bate, A. (2018) *Raising Standards of Infection Prevention and Control in the NHS*. https://commonslibrary.parliament.uk/research-briefings/cdp-2018–0116 (accessed September 7, 2024).

NHS Choices (2021) *How to Wash Your Hands*. https://www.youtube.com/watch?v=d3EPLfzNM_Q (accessed September 7, 2024).

NICE (2014) *Quality Standard 61: Infection Prevention and Control*. https://www.nice.org.uk/guidance/qs61 (accessed September 7, 2024).

NICE (2019 updated 2020) *Surgical Site Infections: Prevention and Treatment*. https://www.nice.org.uk/guidance/ng125 (accessed September 7, 2024).

NICE (2023) *Health-Care Associated Infections*. https://cks.nice.org.uk/topics/healthcare-associated-infections (accessed September 7, 2024).

NMC (2024) *The Code*. https://www.nmc.org.uk/standards/code (accessed September 7, 2024).

Over, P. (2023) *Hand hygiene in the spotlight*. https://www.initial.co.uk/blog/hand-hygiene-in-the-spotlight (accessed November 25, 2024).

RCN (2017) *Essential Practice for Infection Prevention and Control*. https://www.rcn.org.uk/Professional-Development/publications/pub-005940 (accessed September 7, 2024).

Skills for Health (2022) *Perform Hand Hygiene to Prevent the Spread of Infection*. https://tools.skillsforhealth.org.uk/competence-details/html/4622 (accessed September 11, 2024).

Teare, L., Cookson, B., and Stone, S. (2001) Hand hygiene. *BMJ* 323: 411–412. https://www.bmj.com/content/323/7310/411.short (accessed October 28, 2024).

World Health Organisation WHO (2009a) *Your 5 Moments for Hand Hygiene* (Poster). https://cdn.who.int/media/docs/default-source/integrated-health-services-(ihs)/infection-prevention-and-control/your-5-moments-for-hand-hygiene-poster.pdf (accessed September 7, 2024).

World Health Organisation WHO (2009b) *WHO Guidelines on Hand Hygiene in Health Care*. https://www.ncbi.nlm.nih.gov/books/NBK144013 (accessed September 7, 2024).

Chaperoning

11

In recent years, the role of the chaperone in healthcare has been recognised as increasingly important for patients and healthcare providers alike. It is often performed badly, leaving the health professional and patient open to abuse, and so it is vital that all those who are to perform the role understand the reason for it and can do it properly. This chapter will outline the history behind the current situation and will provide guidelines for healthcare workers who may be asked to perform this role in the future.

All healthcare professionals have become acutely aware of the need to protect themselves from allegations of **malpractice** in today's litigious society. Furthermore, it has become clear that the title of 'doctor' or 'nurse' does not always guarantee protection for the patient. Consider the case of Harold Shipman, who was a GP who murdered more than 200 patients (Smith 2003). Consider also the case of Jimmy Savile, who so blatantly abused his position of trust as a hospital porter and used his status as a respected fundraising celebrity to abuse children and vulnerable patients for many decades. It is an unfortunate fact of life that in any sector of society, there will be people who will choose to abuse their positions of trust and respect to satisfy their own perverse needs. Baker (2004), writing about Shipman, argues that systems to protect the public and regulate the professions have been inadequate.

THE AYLING INQUIRY

In 2004, the Department of Health (now Department of Health and Social Care) set up an independent investigation into how the NHS handled allegations about the conduct of GP Clifford Ayling (DoH 2004). He was convicted of 13 counts of indecent assault on patients between 1991 and 1998. The report describes a 'long history of continuing unease' regarding the GP's behaviour, which was overfamiliar and unprofessional when performing intimate examinations. His colleagues appear to have ignored the warning signs and 'reworked the truth' to make it more acceptable, and had ultimately failed their patients. This investigation culminated in

DOI: 10.4324/9781003460381-14

the Ayling Inquiry of 2004, and it is this that has been the **catalyst** for the increased awareness of the importance of the role of the chaperone. The report recommended that all patients should be offered a chaperone for intimate examinations, and that each NHS trust should create a chaperone policy, make it explicit to patients and resource it accordingly. In spite of this, it seems likely that the use of chaperones is still afforded only a low priority although many NHS trusts in England have now implemented a chaperone policy. A study into GPs performing pelvic examinations in women identified several problems with the use of chaperones (Williams et al. 2023). While most of the 14 GPs interviewed offered a chaperone, some did not and some felt it made the examination more awkward. One male GP felt the need for a chaperone in an older woman was less than with a younger woman. Only one of the GP participants described the benefit of a chaperone for a very nervous patient. Lack of suitable staff was also identified as a barrier to the use of chaperones. This was obviously a very small study, but it is interesting nevertheless.

WHAT IS A CHAPERONE?

There is no established single definition of the term chaperone. It originates from the fifteenth century, when it meant 'hood for a hawk', and later came to mean 'a woman who protects a young single woman'. In French, the word 'chaperonner' means to cover with a hood, and today the word is used in the sense of 'protector' (Wai et al. 2008).

A Medical Protection fact sheet (Medical Protection 2020) defines the term 'chaperone' as 'an impartial observer present during an intimate examination of a patient'. It goes on to stress that 'The chaperone should usually be a health professional who has been appropriately trained for the role and who is familiar with the procedure involved'.

The chaperone can act as an advocate for the patient, assessing their understanding and offering an explanation when necessary. However, no matter how good the chaperone is, this does not negate the need for good communication and an adequate explanation of the procedure by the health professional performing the examination.

When is a chaperone needed?

The most common reasons for needing a chaperone are the following.

- To offer the patient protection against verbal, physical or sexual abuse, and to identify inappropriate behaviour.

- To add a layer of protection for the health worker against allegations of malpractice. A chaperone cannot be a guarantee of protection for either the examiner or examinee, but it is very rare for an allegation of assault to be made if a chaperone is present (Medical Protection 2023).
- To support the patient by providing reassurance and physical and emotional comfort during an embarrassing 'sensitive' examination.
- To maintain the patient's dignity and self-respect.
- When the patient requests a chaperone.
- When the doctor feels that a chaperone is necessary.

This list is not exhaustive, and the Medical Defence Union has produced fictional scenarios to demonstrate how a chaperone may be needed in other situations such as where dim lighting is required or where the health worker needs to get very close to the patient, for example during otoscopy (examining the ears with an otoscope) or ophthalmoscopy (examining the eyes) (Simpson 2010).

A 'sensitive' examination may denote one that involves examining the breasts, rectum or genitalia, but it could be used to describe any part of the body depending on the religion and cultural customs of the patient. Some authors argue that examination of the torso should also routinely be considered under the heading of intimate examination, as cases of inappropriate behaviour during such examinations have generated huge concern (Wai et al. 2008).

Other situations when chaperones may be beneficial have been outlined by Medical Protection (2023) and include those when there are vulnerable or anxious patients, patients with whom there may have been a difficulty or misunderstanding in the past, or patients being seen by trainee doctors or students.

What if a patient declines to have a chaperone?

It is important to document that the offer was made and declined. The health worker should explain that they would prefer a chaperone to be present and explain the role of the chaperone. They should explore the reasons why the patient doesn't want a chaperone and address any concerns they may have. The healthcare professional may decline to examine the patient in this case if, in their clinical judgement, this would put them at risk of unjust or invalid accusation.

Chaperone policy

There should be a chaperone policy in place so that all members of the team understand what the role entails. The policy should be clearly advertised in the surgery through patient information leaflets, websites and notice boards. You, as the HCA, may be the best person to prepare an information poster for the waiting areas. The poster should outline the role and availability of chaperones and how patients can request one. Clear notices will reassure patients and increase understanding regarding the need of either doctor or patient to expect an extra degree of protection.

The HCA as chaperone

Before the Ayling Inquiry (DoH 2004), there were very few, if any, recommendations as to who should act as a chaperone, and it would usually have been the nurse or female receptionist who were expected to perform the role. Friends or relatives may also have been used as chaperones, but are no longer considered appropriate. For patients with learning difficulties, a family member or carer may be present to support the patient, and in this instance a careful and sensitive explanation of the procedure is vital.

As an HCA, the role of chaperone will be one you can perform very competently, providing you have the appropriate training.

As a member of the clinical staff, you will usually have had a Disclosure and Barring Service (DBS) check, but when non-clinical staff are used for this role, they will need to have a DBS check depending on their specific duties as chaperone and the contact they have with patients, especially children and vulnerable adults (CQC 2024).

Remember that as an HCA, you might need to have a chaperone yourself for some procedures. For example, when performing an electrocardiograph (ECG), you may need a chaperone, particularly if you are a male HCA and your patient is female, or when performing a wound dressing when clothing must be removed.

Men appear to be unfairly discriminated against when having an intimate examination because most chaperones are female. There should (ideally) be men available in the practice who can chaperone male patients if required, but this obviously won't always be possible.

Chaperoning the gay or transgender patient

Remember, gay patients may prefer a chaperone of the opposite gender. All patients should be able to choose the gender of their chaperone if possible. Take care to use preferred gender titles with transgender patients.

CHAPERONING: THE PROCEDURE

1. Introduce yourself to the patient.
2. Check that they have consented to your presence.
3. Give the patient privacy to undress and provide a dignity sheet to preserve their dignity.
4. Do not assist the patient with the removal of their clothes unless they indicate that they need assistance.
5. Assist the patient on to the examining couch only when necessary, and without putting yourself at risk of injury.
6. Only expose the area of the body required for the doctor to carry out the examination.
7. Maintain a position whereby you can observe the procedure throughout. This means you should always stand *inside* the curtains and usually at the head of the couch.
8. Check that the doctor has explained the procedure and that the patient understands what the examination will involve.
9. Keep the discussion relevant to the procedure and avoid unnecessary personal comments. Although it is sometimes tempting to discuss the weather or other topics to try to relax the patient, this can have the effect of distracting the patient and chaperone, and may make it more difficult for the patient to voice any concerns or discomfort.
10. Ensure that the patient's dignity and privacy are respected as far as possible throughout the procedure.

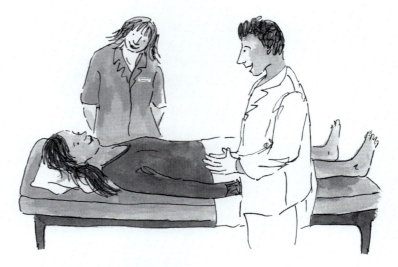

Figure 11.1 HCA chaperoning

11 Check for continuing consent if the patient appears to be uncomfortable or unhappy.
12 At the end of the examination, allow the patient privacy to redress fully, and only leave the room when they are fully dressed and before the doctor continues with the consultation.
13 Remember to observe infection control guidelines throughout.
14 Observe strict confidentiality, and do not discuss the consultation or examination with any other members of staff except on a 'need to know' basis. If you have any concerns about the procedure, always discuss these with your nurse mentor and document them clearly.
15 The healthcare professional should document details of the examination, including the presence (or absence) of a chaperone and their name and the information given. They should also document any reservations or concerns the patient or they themselves may have had.

ACTIVITY

Consider the following scenario.

The doctor has asked you to act as chaperone for him to perform a breast examination. When you go into the room, you realise that the patient is someone you know quite well, and she appears quite nervous and flustered when she sees you.

Dr Jones quickly introduces you to the patient (Mrs X) and asks you to stand just inside the curtain at the foot of the bed. Mrs X takes off her blouse, as instructed by the doctor, but has some difficulty with the buttons, so you help her. You make some small talk to try to relax her as she seems very tense – you ask about her children and chat about the recent bad weather. You also admire her all-over tan, all the time trying to relax Mrs X.

Dr Jones comes behind the curtain and stands between you and the patient. He asks Mrs X to remove her bra and then proceeds to study her two breasts intently. He then asks Mrs X to raise her hands above her head and then to put her hands on her hips, all the while staring at her breasts. You're feeling a little embarrassed by now, so you look the other way and hope Mrs X will notice that you're not staring as well.

Dr Jones then proceeds to feel both Mrs X's breasts, as well as in the armpits and around the neck. Mrs X is looking very red and uncomfortable, and you do find yourself wondering why he needs to be so thorough when she only complained of a lump in one breast. Still, he's the doctor and must know what he's doing.

Chaperoning

> The breast examination given in the scenario is exactly as it should be done, but if this is not explained to the patient, it would seem a little odd.

While examining Mrs X, Dr Jones talks to you, commenting on how busy the surgery is and asking if you will get the notes out for the next patient when you go out.

When Dr Jones has finished examining Mrs X, and before she puts her top back on, he thanks you for your help and suggests that you can now leave. You're glad to get out because you just find the whole thing so awkward.

How do you think the patient would have felt in this scenario, and why?

Using the information given in the chapter, suggest some ways this experience could have been improved for the patient and made safer in terms of protecting the doctor from allegations of malpractice.

TIME TO REFLECT

Using a framework for reflection (see Chapter 2), try reflecting on a consultation when you were acting as a chaperone, or alternatively where you have been chaperoned as a patient yourself.

How did it go, and what did you learn?

REFERENCES

Baker, R (2004) Patient-centred care after Shipman. *Journal of the Royal Society of Medicine* 97(4): 161–165. https://www.ncbi.nlm.nih.gov/pmc/articles/PMC1079351/ (accessed September 11, 2024).

CQC (2024) *GP Mythbuster 15: Chaperones*. https://www.cqc.org.uk/guidance-providers/gps/gp-mythbusters/gp-mythbuster-15-chaperones (accessed September 11, 2024).

Department of Health DoH (2004) *Committee of Inquiry: Independent Investigation into How the NHS Handled Allegations About the Conduct of Clifford Ayling*. https://webarchive.nationalarchives.gov.uk/ukgwa/+/http://www.dh.gov.uk/en/Publicationsandstatistics/Publications/PublicationsPolicyAndGuidance/DH_4088996 (accessed September 11, 2024).

Medical Protection (2020) *Chaperones*. https://www.medicalprotection.org/uk/articles/chaperones (accessed September 11, 2024).

Medical Protection (2023) *Chaperones*. https://www.medicalprotection.org/ireland/resources-training/factsheets/factsheets/roi-chaperones (accessed September 11, 2024).

Simpson, B. (2010) *Gponline. Medico-Legal – The Essential role of Chaperones*. https://www.gponline.com/medico-legal-essential-role-chaperones/article/995942

Smith, J. (2003) *The Shipman Inquiry*. https://assets.publishing.service.gov.uk/government/uploads/system/uploads/attachment_data/file/273227/5854.pdf (accessed September 11, 2024).

Wai, D., Keighley, B., Hendry, R., et al. (2008) Chaperones: Are we protecting patients? *British Journal of General Practice* 58(546): 54–57. https://pubmed.ncbi.nlm.nih.gov/18187001 (accessed October 28, 2024).

Williams, P., Murchie, P., Cruikshank, E., Bond, C., and Burton, D. (2023) What influences GPs' use of pelvic examination? A qualitative investigation in primary care. *British Journal of General Practice* 73(732). https://doi.org/10.3399/BJGP.2022.0363 (accessed May 14, 2024).

Section III
Core skills

Chapter 12	Physiological measurements	111
Chapter 13	Understanding and measuring blood pressure accurately	125
Chapter 14	Understanding the heart: How to perform the electrocardiograph (ECG)	135
Chapter 15	Venepuncture and capillary blood testing: best practice	149
Chapter 16	Kidney function and urine: performing accurate urinalysis	167

Physiological measurements

12

Whenever performing any physiological measurement, always inform the patient fully, explaining what the procedure involves, and make sure that you have consent to proceed.

Decontaminate your hands before and after patient contact.

You can download the National Occupational Standard SFHCHS19 *Undertake Routine Clinical Measurements* to use as a checklist for your competencies (Skills for Health 2021).

HEIGHT, WEIGHT, BODY MASS INDEX (BMI) AND WAIST MEASUREMENT

BMI = weight in kilograms/height in metres
(most computers will calculate this automatically)

Why do we record weight, height and BMI?

Recording a patient's BMI can be useful to help identify those people who are overweight or underweight, and at increased risk of the associated health problems (see Box 12.1).

Box 12.1 Why check the BMI?

- To monitor normal growth in children.
- To check for abnormal loss of weight, for example in malnutrition, malignancy or alcoholism.
- To check for abnormal loss of height, for example in osteoporosis when the spine crumbles.
- To enable the doctor to prescribe certain medications or therapies when the dose is dependent on the patient's weight.
- To enable accurate measurement of lung function.
- To encourage patients who are trying to lose or gain weight.

BMI: good or bad?

NICE (2024) has produced a classification table to demonstrate the meaning of BMI measurements in relation to a healthy weight and obesity (see Table 12.1).

Table 12.1 Obesity: classification

Classification	BMI
Healthy weight	18.5–24.9
Overweight	25.0–29.9
Obesity 1	30.0–34.9
Obesity 2	35.0–39.9
Obesity 3	40.0+

While BMI is useful, it is not always an accurate indicator of health. The two men in Figure 12.1 have the same BMI, but which one do you think has the greatest health risk?

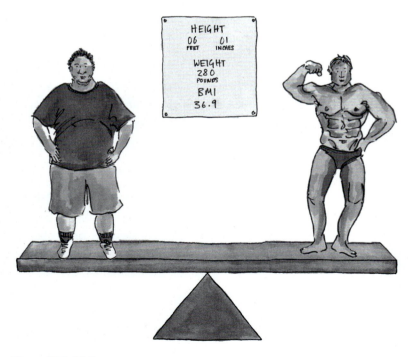

Figure 12.1 BMI

Physiological measurements

Remember, muscle weighs more than fat, so if a person is very fit and has built up a lot of muscle, this can render the BMI useless as a determinant of health.

Central adiposity, whereby fat is laid down more around the middle (commonly referred to as the 'apple shape') is also an important factor and carries a greater risk of health problems such as Type 2 diabetes or heart disease than those people who have a 'pear shape', with larger buttocks and thighs. This is because the type of fat that tends to accumulate around the abdomen appears to block the effect of insulin on the cells, making it harder for the cells to take in glucose. This is thought to create **insulin resistance** so that the body responds by producing more glucose, which may eventually result in Type 2 diabetes. This theory has previously been controversial, but more recent research has provided new evidence that supports the original theory and shows a clear correlation between the 'apple shape' and insulin resistance (Shungin et al. 2015), as well as a link with an increased risk of myocardial infarction, particularly in women (Peters et al. 2018). Because of this, the NICE (2024) guidelines also advise consideration of ethnicity and the use of lower BMI levels to determine obesity in people with a South Asian, Chinese, other Asian, Middle Eastern, Black African or African Caribbean family background, as they are prone to central obesity and their cardiometabolic risk occurs at a lower BMI.

Considering the importance of central adiposity, it makes sense to measure the waist in conjunction with the BMI and this is currently considered to be best practice, and more useful as an indicator of risk (see Table 12.2).

Table 12.2 Obesity: risk assessment with waist measurement

BMI classification	Waist circumference		
	Low	High	Very high
Overweight	No increased risk	Increased risk	High risk
Obesity 1	Increased risk	High risk	Very high risk
For men, waist circumference of less than 94 cm is low, 94–102 cm is high, and more than 102 cm is very high. For women, waist circumference of less than 80 cm is low, 80–88 cm is high, and more than 88 cm is very high			

RECORDING HEIGHT, WEIGHT AND WAIST: THE PROCEDURE

Measuring height

Make sure that the height chart/measure has been attached to the wall at the correct height.

Ask the patient to:

- remove their shoes;
- stand upright and look straight ahead; and
- keep heels together, and keep heels, calves, buttocks and back in contact with the wall if possible.

Measure the patient's height to the nearest centimetre.

Measuring weight

Use appropriate medical scales for the task. Recommendations for the types of scales to be used are available online (Best 2020). Using inaccurate equipment may result in errors in diagnosis and treatment (LACORS 2009; see Box 12.2).

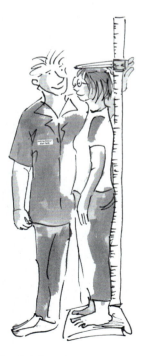

Figure 12.2 HCA measuring height

Box 12.2 Risks associated with inaccurate weight measurement

> A series of pilot studies in 2007 found some staff using inaccurate or unsuitable weighing scales to calculate doses of medication or radiation for some patients, including small children. Following this, The National Medical Weighing Project was set up and made a series of recommendations regarding suitable weighing devices LACORS (2009).

Did you know?

Measurements on analogue scales can be increased by as much as 10–12% if the scales are on a soft carpeted surface. Digital scales are less prone to this effect (Pendergast 2002).

Make sure the scales have been calibrated within the last year (or in line with local policy), are on a hard surface and set to zero. Ask the patient to:

- remove outer clothing and shoes; and
- stand squarely on the scales (or sit squarely with feet not touching the floor surface, if using chair scales).

Record the patient's weight to the nearest 0.5kg.

Measuring the waist

- Using a suitable measuring tape that is designed for the purpose, measure directly over skin or over only one item of light clothing.

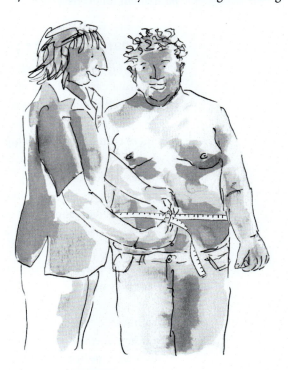

Figure 12.3 HCA measuring waist

- Ask the patient to breathe out normally.
- Hold the tape snugly (without compressing the skin) around the waist, halfway between the lowest rib and the top of the hip bone (roughly in line with or slightly above the belly button).

ACTIVITY

Now measure your own waist.

How do you score on the risk table (see Table 12.2)?

THE PULSE

When the heart contracts, it pushes blood out through the elastic walled arteries. This is felt at various points of the body as a *pulse*; if the arteries are in good condition, the pulse should usually be felt at the same time as the heartbeat. The normal pulse rate is between 60 and 80 beats per minute, but can vary enormously from as low as 40bpm during sleep up to 220bpm or more during strenuous exercise.

An **arrhythmia** is an abnormal rate or rhythm of the heartbeat. Some are more serious than others. Some are intermittent and some will become permanent unless treated.

What can affect the pulse?

It may be *higher* than normal (*tachycardia* = heart rate above 100bpm). Tachycardia can be classified as sinus, ventricular or supraventricular, and there will be different causes for each type. It can occur:

- if there is an infection or a high temperature (pyrexia);
- when the patient is anxious;
- after exercise;
- after stimulants such as coffee or cigarettes;
- in some medical conditions such as **hyperthyroidism**; and
- with some medication, such as adrenaline and salbutamol.

It may also be *lower* than normal (*bradycardia* = heart rate below 50bpm), and this may occur:

- in athletes;
- in some medical conditions, such as hypothyroidism, myocardial infarction, **pericardial tamponade**, **adrenal insufficiency** and **sick sinus syndrome**;

- with some medication, such as beta blockers, digoxin, calcium channel blockers, amiodarone, clonidine and verapamil;
- in **hypoxia**; and
- in hypothermia.

Or it may be *irregular*, without normal rhythm. This can occur in normal healthy hearts, but may also occur:

- in some types of heart disease, such as **atrial fibrillation**;
- where there is an **electrolyte** imbalance;
- if there are changes in heart muscle; and
- if there is injury from a myocardial infarction (heart attack).

Pulse amplitude refers to the strength of the pulse and the elasticity of the artery wall. A pulse may be described as strong or 'bounding', which may indicate infection. Or it may be weak, faint or 'thready', which may signify shock or hypovolaemia (low fluid levels).

RECORDING THE RADIAL OR BRACHIAL PULSE: THE PROCEDURE

1. Use two fingers, and press quite firmly over the area at the base of the thumb for the radial pulse (see Figure 12.5) and on the inside of the elbow for the brachial pulse (see Figure 12.6).

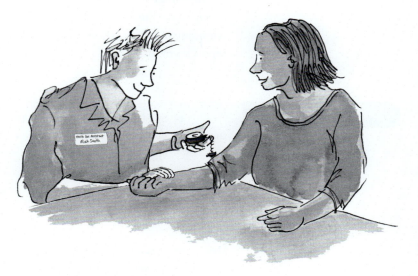

Figure 12.4 HCA taking pulse at wrist

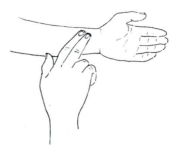

Figure 12.5 Radial pulse

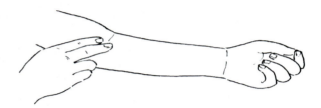

Figure 12.6 Brachial pulse

2 Record the rate by counting how many beats there are in 30 seconds, then multiply this figure by two to record the beats per minute.
3 If the pulse is irregular, you will need to measure it for a full minute.
4 Document the result immediately, and always check with the doctor or nurse if the pulse seems very fast or slow or is irregular. You may also notice if the pulse seems unusually weak or is very strong or bounding in nature. These may be important observations, so always report them.

> **ACTIVITY**
>
> Draw a body outline and see if you can mark where all the various pulses can be found. Check your answers against Figure 12.7.
> Using Figures 12.5 and 12.6 for guidance, see if you can you find your own pulses in the wrist (radial pulse) and inside the elbow (brachial pulse).

Measuring a pulse with a **Doppler** can be useful in patients who have or are at risk of arterial disease, but specific training is required to use the Doppler correctly.

Physiological measurements

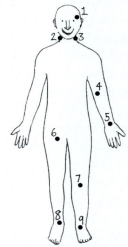

Figure 12.7 Pulse points

RESPIRATORY RATE

The respiratory rate is a key vital sign, and it is used to detect early changes when monitoring very ill patients.

We breathe in oxygen (required to produce energy) and breathe out carbon dioxide (a waste product of metabolism), and most of us will breathe at a rate of about 12–20 breaths per minute. It is an essential but subconscious mechanism, and we only become aware of it when it becomes difficult or if we know we are being observed.

The respiratory rate may be affected by:

- exercise;
- stress and emotion;
- illness; and
- some medication.

A rate of less than 12 breaths per minute or more than 25 breaths per minute is considered abnormal (in adults).

Recording the respiratory rate: the procedure

1 *Look*. Is the patient distressed? Can they complete a sentence without stopping for breath? Are there any signs of **cyanosis** (for example, a

blue colour around the lips)? Whenever you are unsure, always refer the patient back to the doctor or nurse.

2 *Note how the patient breathes*, as well as the rate. A person who has difficulty breathing will be using all their accessory muscles, sometimes lifting their shoulders up and down to help the lungs expand. There may be intercostal recession (sucking in of the skin between the ribs), which is one of the key signs of respiratory distress. Some patients will also breathe out through pursed lips. This is very typical of patients with chronic obstructive pulmonary disease (COPD), and is a method of trying to expel all the carbon dioxide slowly. Rapid expiration is more likely to force the diseased airways to collapse.

3 *Listen to the breathing.* Is there an audible wheeze or other abnormal noise?

4 *Recording a patient's respiratory rate* can be difficult because the rate will change if the patient knows they are being observed. Because of this, it is better to count the breaths per minute when holding the wrist as if still checking the pulse rate, so that the patient is unaware. As with measuring the pulse, you should count for 30 seconds and multiply by two to achieve the rate per minute. If the patient is breathing irregularly, you will need to count for a full minute.

PULSE OXIMETRY

A pulse oximeter provides a non-invasive method of measuring the oxygenation of a patient's blood. It works by shining an infrared light through the tissues of the body and detecting the colour difference between oxygenated and unoxygenated blood.

A beam of infrared light is passed through the chosen area, and the degree of absorption will depend on the amount of oxygen in the blood. Pulse oximeters will often give a reading of the pulse rate, as well.

Pulse oximetry is used routinely in intensive care, operating theatres and recovery rooms.

It may be used in a doctor's surgery to monitor a patient's oxygen levels when they are having respiratory difficulty, such as during an asthma attack or worsening COPD or during a heart attack. Some patients who are receiving medication that may depress their respiration, such as strong **opiate analgesics**, may also need to have their oxygen levels monitored.

Accuracy can be affected by the thickness and temperature of the skin, so it is important to place the sensor in the best possible place. This will normally be on an area where the skin is relatively thin, such as the

Physiological measurements

fingertip or earlobe. Other factors – such as nail varnish, dirt, foreign objects or bright lighting – can affect the light transmission, and therefore give erroneous results. Pulse detection may be affected by excessive movement, shivering, poor circulation and atrial fibrillation.

The normal level for oxygen saturation of the blood is between 96% and 100%. Levels below 90% can be life-threatening.

Recording pulse oximetry: the procedure

1 Ensure the patient is comfortable and warm enough.
2 Select a suitable site, such as the fingertip, and make sure that any nail varnish, dirt, etc., has been removed. Choose a finger where the skin is not callused or thickened.
3 Place the probe according to the manufacturer's instructions.
4 Make sure the sensor is also detecting the pulse.
5 Make a note of the oxygen level and remove the probe.
6 Clean and store the probe according to the manufacturer's instructions.
7 Document the reading and report any abnormal oxygen levels.

TEMPERATURE

You need to know the following terms.

- *Apyrexial*: Normal temperature. Usually considered to be a range anywhere between 36.2°C and 37.7°C.
- *Pyrexia*: High temperature. May also be referred to as a fever, and less commonly referred to as hyperthermia.
- *Hypothermia*: Low temperature. We feel cold if our core temperature is 36°C, start to shiver at 35°C, become clumsy and confused at 34°C, develop muscle stiffness at 32°C, and at 28°C would be at risk of cardiac arrest.

The temperature may be taken to check for an infection anywhere in the body when a patient is feeling unwell. It will also be checked routinely post-operatively to make sure a patient is not developing an infection. Patients with surgical wounds are more susceptible to infection, which can then delay healing.

When you consider the potential implications of an infection for any person, the importance of measuring the temperature accurately cannot be overemphasised. There are various devices for checking temperature, but the one used most commonly (and often incorrectly) is the tympanic thermometer. This uses an infrared light to detect the temperature at the tympanic membrane (eardrum).

Recording the temperature: the procedure

Always check the manufacturer's instructions for use, as the devices may vary slightly.

1. Place a disposable cap over the nozzle of the thermometer.
2. Press the button to turn it on, and then place the nozzle just inside the ear canal and point it forwards.
3. Depress the button until a beep is heard, then gently withdraw the nozzle and note the temperature displayed.
4. Remember, the device must be placed just *inside* the ear canal, pointing towards the tympanic membrane, to take an accurate reading.
5. Report any temperature that falls outside the normal parameters to the doctor or nurse.

Other devices to check the temperature may be used in some settings, including the following.

- A rectal thermometer provides the most reliable core temperature, but is obviously the most invasive and least 'user-friendly'!
- Oral digital thermometers that can be placed inside the cheek (buccal) or under the tongue (sublingual) can be used, but must be held in place for long enough, and will give a reading that is slightly lower than core body temperature.
- Body surface thermometers are placed in the **axilla** or groin, but again will need to be held there for long enough, and may give a significantly lower result than the actual core body temperature.
- Forehead thermometers are the least intrusive, and can be useful for babies and toddlers.

Now try the following quiz. You can check back in the text for the answers.

PHYSIOLOGICAL MEASUREMENTS QUIZ

1. How do you calculate the BMI?
2. When does the BMI indicate a person is overweight?

Physiological measurements

3   Why is it useful to measure the waist as well as the BMI?
4   If a woman is overweight according to her BMI and her waist measurement is 78 cm, is she at increased risk of health problems or not?
5   What is the normal pulse rate for an adult?
6   Where would you find the brachial pulse?
7   What is the normal respiratory rate for an adult?
8   List two factors that can affect the accuracy of the pulse oximetry reading.
9   What is the normal level for oxygen saturation of the blood?
10 What is the normal range for body temperature?

TIME TO REFLECT

Using a framework for reflection (see Chapter 2), try reflecting on a consultation when you performed a physiological measurement.

How did it go and what have you learnt?

REFERENCES

Best, C. (2020) *Accurate Measurement of Weight and Height 1: Weighing Patients.* https://cdn.ps.emap.com/wp-content/uploads/sites/3/2020/03/200325-Accurate-measurement-of-weight-and-height-1-weighing-patients.pdf (accessed September 13, 2024).

Local Authority Coordinators of Regulatory Services LACORS (2009) *The Weight of the Matter: Final Report of the LACORS National Medical Weighing Project 2008/2009.* https://metricviews.uk/wp-content/uploads/2023/04/21749.pdf (accessed September 13, 2024).

NICE (2024) *How Should I Confirm if a Person is Overweight or Obese?* https://cks.nice.org.uk/topics/obesity/diagnosis/identification-classification (accessed September 11, 2024).

Pendergast, J. (2002) *Why You Weigh More on Thick Carpet.* http://www.inference.phy.cam.ac.uk/is/papers/bathroom_scales.pdf (accessed September 7, 2024).

Peters, S., Bots, S., and Woodward, M. (2018) Sex differences in the association between measures of general and central adiposity and the risk of myocardial infarction: Results from the UK Biobank. *Journal of the American Heart Association* 7(5). https://www.ncbi.nlm.nih.gov/pubmed/29490971 (accessed September 11, 2024).

Shungin, D., Winkler, T., Croteau-Chonka, D. et al. (2015) New genetic loci link adipose and insulin biology to body fat distribution. *Nature*

518: 187–196. https://www.nature.com/articles/nature14132?WT.ec_id=NATURE-20150212 (accessed September 11, 2024).

Skills for Health (2021) *CHS19 Undertake Routine Clinical Measurements*. https://tools.skillsforhealth.org.uk/competence-details/html/4371 (accessed September 13, 2024).

Understanding and measuring blood pressure accurately

13

Measuring and recording blood pressure is an important task that is often delegated to the HCA. Before you learn how to perform this task, it is essential that you understand *what* you are doing and *why*. Only then can you learn how to make an accurate measurement and understand why it is so important.

WHAT IS BLOOD PRESSURE?

Arteries are the blood vessels that carry blood away from the heart. Every time the heart contracts, it squeezes blood through the arteries and the blood exerts a force on the artery walls. This force is the *blood pressure*.

Human blood pressure was first recorded in 1847 by Carl Ludwig, who inserted a catheter into a patient's artery and connected the catheter to an invention called a kymograph. In 1896, the mercury-filled sphygmoma-nometer was developed by Scipione Riva-Rocci, and blood pressure was measured according to how high the pressure could lift a column of mercury (Roguin 2006). We still refer to the measurement in millimetres of mercury (known by its chemical symbol of Hg).

The *systolic pressure* measures the force exerted by the blood on the artery walls at the peak of the left ventricular contraction. The left ventricle is the largest chamber in the heart (for more detail on heart anatomy, see Chapter 14). The systolic pressure is the higher of the two readings.

The *diastolic pressure* measures the force exerted on the artery walls when the heart is relaxed.

The pressure in the arteries will depend on how hard the heart is pumping and how much resistance there is in the arteries.

There are several things that will create an increase in the resistance in the artery.

> The word *diastolic* sounds more relaxed than *systolic* – this is a good way to remember the difference. You could also think of **d**iastolic as referring to the **d**ownbeat phase.

- If the diameter of the artery is reduced, as for example in atherosclerosis, where there are fatty deposits sticking to the artery walls.
- If the walls of the artery are stiff or rigid. Think of an old hosepipe compared with a new one. In the new piece of hose, the walls are more elastic

DOI: 10.4324/9781003460381-17

and stretchy. The pressure can be absorbed as the wall stretches, whereas the pressure will be greater in the rigid hose. As arteries age, they become stiffer, so blood pressure will invariably increase a little with age.

- If the blood is thicker or stickier than normal. This can happen when the number of red blood cells increases in a condition called **polycythaemia**. Red blood cells carry oxygen, so patients who have problems taking on enough oxygen (such as those with respiratory disease) may adapt by producing more red blood cells. Smokers may also have this problem.
- If the volume of blood is increased. Again, imagine what happens when you turn up the tap and force more water through a hose. The volume of blood may be increased in patients who are having **intravenous** fluids or those who are retaining fluid, such as in kidney disease.

WHAT IS HYPERTENSION, AND WHY DOES IT MATTER?

There are two types of hypertension:

- *essential hypertension*, when the cause is not known; and
- *secondary hypertension*, which may be due to medication (e.g. combined contraceptive pill, steroids), kidney disease or hormone problems.

A patient may be diagnosed with hypertension if the blood pressure measurements show an isolated high systolic pressure (e.g. 180/70) or an isolated high diastolic pressure (e.g. 130/100) or both (e.g. 170/110).

Pulse pressure refers to the difference between the systolic and diastolic blood pressures, and this is often increased in older people, who may exhibit normal diastolic readings with isolated systolic hypertension, thought to be due to age-related stiffness of the arteries.

Hypertension can only be diagnosed after several readings (usually a minimum of three) at different times of the day when the patient is relaxed. The phenomenon of white coat hypertension is well known, and refers to how some people will always have a higher blood pressure when they are in a clinical setting, probably due to anxiety (often without the patient realising). Because of this, the current guidelines now suggest that all patients should be offered **ambulatory blood pressure monitoring** (ABPM) or home blood pressure monitoring (HBPM) if they cannot tolerate ABPM (NICE 2019 updated 2023).

These patients will need to have a 24-hour monitor to make an accurate diagnosis or may be advised to purchase a home monitor to perform

Understanding and measuring blood pressure accurately

serial readings at home. In this case, they must be advised to buy a monitor that is validated by the British and Irish Hypertension Society (BIHS) or the British Heart Foundation (BHF) to ensure accuracy. For a list of blood pressure monitors validated for home and specialist (clinical) use, see BIHS (2023) and BIHS (2024).

The home monitor should be checked against the surgery monitor.

There are various grades of hypertension:

- grade 1 (mild hypertension): 140–159/90–99;
- grade 2 (moderate hypertension): 160–179/100–109; and
- grade 3 (severe hypertension): greater than or equal to 180/110.

Do you know when to bring a patient back for further readings and when to refer them to the nurse or doctor? For HCAs who work in primary care, a flow chart based on the NICE guidelines (NICE 2019 updated 2023) is provided in Box 13.1, but you may wish to discuss this with your nurse or doctor and amend it in line with your surgery protocol.

ACTIVITY

How many factors can you think of that might increase your risk of developing high blood pressure and heart disease (see Figure 13.1)?

Check your answers against those given in Box 13.2.

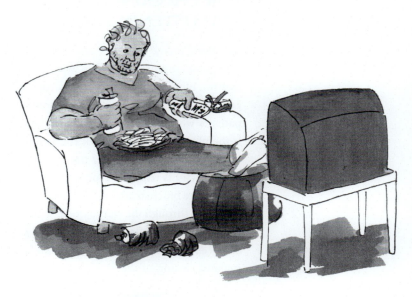

Figure 13.1 An unhealthy lifestyle

SO, WHAT'S ALL THE FUSS ABOUT?

Hypertension is often referred to as 'the silent killer' because it usually has no symptoms, but over time – if left untreated – it can cause strain on the heart and the arteries. It is one of the most important preventable causes of premature heart disease and death in the UK; it is estimated that there are up to 14 million people in the UK with high blood pressure, with five million of these undiagnosed (BHF 2024). There are many possible complications, including angina, heart attacks, **heart failure**, stroke, **peripheral vascular disease**, kidney damage and eye damage. It is often under-diagnosed and inadequately treated.

The role of the HCA in measuring and recording BP *accurately* is therefore vital. When a diagnosis is finally made, it has the following huge implications for the patient and the NHS.

- There is no cure, and patients will need lifelong treatment.
- It is often best controlled by using two or more medications.
- Many treatments cause side effects.
- More tablets mean more potential interactions with other medications.
- There is increased cost to the individual and the NHS.
- Patients require regular monitoring and blood tests.

AUSCULTATORY OR MANUAL METHOD FOR CHECKING THE BP: WHAT ARE YOU LISTENING TO?

Although many surgeries and wards have now disposed of mercury sphygmomanometers in line with European regulations on mercury control, blood pressure is still recorded in mmHg. Many hospital wards and surgeries now use automatic monitors, but these cannot be used on patients who have an irregular heartbeat such as in atrial fibrillation. It is therefore important that all HCAs have the training to enable them to take a blood pressure using the **auscultatory** (listening) method. To do this, the cuff is wrapped around the upper arm and inflated until it compresses the brachial artery. The blood cannot flow through, so no sounds are heard through the stethoscope, which is placed over the artery. Gradually, the cuff is deflated until the blood can just force its way through the artery each time the heart contracts and pushes the blood out. This opening and closing of the artery causes a tapping sound that can be heard through the stethoscope, and this is the systolic pressure. As the cuff is deflated still further, the artery opens and blood flows more easily so that the forced tapping sound muffles or disappears altogether. This change in the sound represents the diastolic pressure when the heart is relaxed. These sounds are called the Korotkoff sounds after the man who discovered them, and there are five possible sounds that can be detected. You usually listen for Korotkoff 1, when the tapping sound begins to denote the systolic pressure, and then for Korotkoff 5, when the sound disappears completely to denote the diastolic pressure. Sometimes the tapping sound may continue, in which case you record Korotkoff 4: the point at which the tapping sound becomes muffled.

MEASURING BLOOD PRESSURE: THE PROCEDURE

You can download the National Occupational Standard CHS19 *Undertake Routine Clinical Measurements* to use as a check list for your competencies (Skills for Health 2021).

1   Explain what you are doing to your patient and why. Make sure you have their informed consent before you continue.

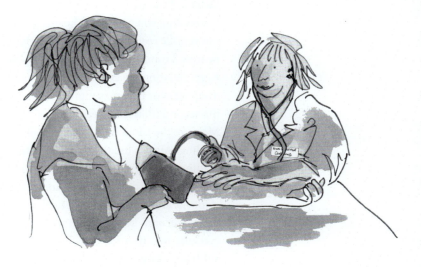

Figure 13.2 Measuring blood pressure

2 Wash or decontaminate your hands before and after the procedure.

3 Make sure the patient is seated comfortably (preferably sitting quietly for five minutes before proceeding). The arm should be free of any constrictive clothing and supported at the level of the heart.

4 Wrap the cuff around the upper arm with the centre of the bladder located over the brachial artery. The cuff must be large enough so that the bladder circles 80% of the arm. In larger patients, a large cuff must be used to avoid the risk of inaccurate high readings.

5 Some teaching resources advocate the idea of positioning the cuff so that the tubing comes from the top. This avoids noise from the tubing bumping against the stethoscope from being confused with the arterial sounds.

6 It is good practice to palpate the brachial or radial pulse and then inflate the cuff until the pulse disappears. Note the readings when the pulse disappears and add 30. Remember this reading. Now deflate the cuff.

7 Position the stethoscope over the brachial artery and reinflate the cuff to the level you noted previously. You should not be able to hear the tapping from the brachial artery. If you can still hear it, inflate the cuff a little more until it disappears.

8 Deflate the cuff very slowly (this takes practice). You should record the reading when you first hear the pulse come back in. This is the systolic reading (Korotkoff 1). This should be recorded to the nearest 2 mm, and never rounded up or down.

9 Keep deflating the cuff very slowly until the tapping sound disappears or becomes muffled (Korotkoff 4 or Korotkoff 5). This is the second (diastolic) reading.

10 Measure the BP in both arms initially and record the highest reading. Always use this arm in the future. If the difference in readings between the arms is 20 mmHg or more, always report this to the nurse or doctor. It may indicate a problem called subclavian stenosis, and should prompt further investigation.

11 Take a second measurement from the chosen arm during the consultation. If this is very different from the first reading, then take a third reading. Record the lower of the last two measurements as the clinic reading.

12 Elderly and diabetic patients may need to have their blood pressure checked again after two minutes standing to check for **postural**

hypotension (a common cause of falls in the elderly). In this case, you should still try to support the arm at the level of the heart so there is no muscular contraction in the arm, as this may interfere with the reading.

13 If using digital/automatic monitors, wrap the cuff around the upper arm as instructed in the monitor guidelines. Make sure the arm is free of restrictive clothing and is supported comfortably at the level of the heart. Press the record button and wait for the cuff to inflate and deflate before making a note of the recording. If the monitor indicates an error (e.g. if the patient has an arrhythmia), the manual method must be used and the nurse or doctor informed.

14 Always discourage the patient from talking during the procedure.

15 Report the readings or recall the patient for further measurements according to your protocol.

16 BP readings must always be recorded using the appropriate read code or template so that they can be easily accessed for future consultations and for audit purposes.

Now try the following quiz. You can check back in the text for the answers.

BLOOD PRESSURE QUIZ

1 What is systolic pressure?
2 List two things that might increase the resistance in the arteries, resulting in a higher blood pressure.
3 Which artery do you place the stethoscope over to listen for the Korotkoff sounds when performing a manual blood pressure measurement?
4 What are the upper limits for systolic and diastolic figures of a normal blood pressure?
5 How many readings are required before hypertension can be diagnosed?
6 If a patient had a blood pressure of 162/98, what would you do?
7 If a patient had blood pressure of 160/110, what would you do?
8 List three complications of hypertension.
9 Which arm should you use to check the blood pressure?
10 What should be offered to the patient whose blood pressure measured in the surgery is equal to or above 140/90, and why?

Box 13.1 Guidelines for HCAs for the referral of patients according to BP

>179 >109	160–179 100–109	140–159 90–99	135–139 85–89	<135 <85
Refer to the doctor on the same day	Recheck three times over next two weeks, then make an appointment with the doctor	Reassess three times weekly, then make an appointment with the doctor	Lifestyle advice, and reassess annually if not on treatment, or in six months if on treatment	Lifestyle advice, and reassess in five years if not on treatment, or in six months if on treatment

All patients whose BP is equal to/above 140/90 should be offered ABPM, or HBPM if ABPM is declined or not tolerated (NICE 2019 updated 2023).

Box 13.2 Risk factors for developing high blood pressure and heart disease

- Poor diet, high in fat or salt.
- High cholesterol, high low-density lipoprotein (LDL), high triglycerides, low high-density lipoprotein (HDL).
- Atheromatous arteries.
- Male gender.
- High levels of alcohol.
- Obesity.
- Lack of exercise.
- Increasing age.
- Diabetes.
- Ethnic group.
- Family history.
- Smoking (although links with sustained hypertension have yet to be established).

TIME TO REFLECT

Using a framework for reflection (see Chapter 2), try reflecting on a consultation when you performed a blood pressure measurement. How did it go, and what did you learn?

How does a blood pressure monitor like to make jokes? Off the cuff!

REFERENCES

BHF (2024) *6 Things You Need to Know About High Blood Pressure*. https://www.bhf.org.uk/informationsupport/heart-matters-magazine/medical/6-things-you-need-to-know-about-high-blood-pressure (accessed September 13, 2024).

British and Irish Hypertension Society [BIHS] (2024) *Validated BP Monitors for Home Use*. https://bihsoc.org/wp-content/uploads/2024/04/Validated-BP-Monitors-For-Home-Use-British-and-Irish-Hypertension-Society.pdf (accessed June 7, 2024).

British and Irish Hypertension Society [BIHS] (2023) *Validated BP Monitors for Specialist Use*. https://bihsoc.org/wp-content/uploads/2023/12/Validated-BP-Monitors-For-Specialist-Use-British-and-Irish-Hypertension-Society–2.pdf (accessed September 13, 2024).

NICE (2019 updated 2023) *Hypertension in Adults: Diagnosis and Management*. https://www.nice.org.uk/guidance/ng136/resources/hypertension-in-adults-diagnosis-and-management-pdf-66141722710213 (accessed September 13, 2024).

Roguin, A. (2006) Scipione Riva-Rocci and the men behind the mercury sphygmanometer. *International Journal of Clinical Practice* 60(1): 73–79. https://pubmed.ncbi.nlm.nih.gov/16409431 (accessed September 7, 2024).

Skills for Health (2021) *CHS19 Undertake Routine Clinical Measurements*. https://tools.skillsforhealth.org.uk/competence-details/html/4371 (accessed September 13, 2024).

Understanding the heart

How to perform the electrocardiograph (ECG)

14

HISTORY OF THE ECG

In the nineteenth century, it became clear that the heart generated electricity. In 1924, Willem Einthoven discovered the electrocardiographic features of the heart and realised that these could be used to detect abnormalities. He assigned the letters PQRST to the various deflections, and was awarded the Nobel Prize for his discovery.

Before you can understand an ECG or how to perform the test accurately, you need to have a basic understanding of the heart and how it works.

WHAT DOES THE HEART DO?

- It is a dual muscular pump. The right and left side of the heart are separated by the septum.
- It squeezes blood through one-way valves in a network of narrowing arteries to the lungs and the rest of the body (see Figure 14.1).
- The heart rate for an average male is between 60 and 80 beats per minute.
- It beats approximately 100,000 times per day (2,920,000,000 times in an average lifespan of 80 years).
- If it stops for just a few seconds, all hell breaks loose!

HEART ANATOMY

The heart has four chambers, the right and left atria and the right and left ventricles (see Figure 14.2).

The arteries carry blood away from the heart, and the veins bring blood back to the heart (remember, artery begins with 'a' for 'away'!). The arteries are therefore under greater pressure and have thicker walls. You will also feel a pulse in the arteries corresponding with the heartbeat, but you will not be able to feel a pulse in a vein. This is because the pressure has

DOI: 10.4324/9781003460381-18

135

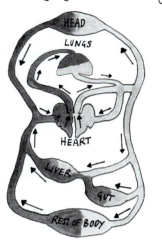

Figure 14.1 Circulatory system

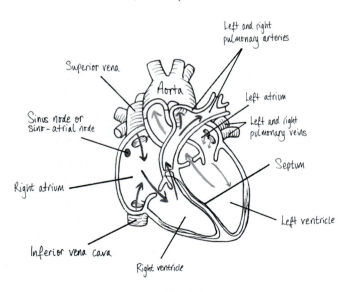

Figure 14.2 Heart anatomy showing blood flow

dropped by the time the blood has travelled through the circulatory system from the heart via arteries to **arterioles**, then to **capillaries** and then to **venuoles**, before being transported back to the heart via the veins.

Blood that has been around the body and exhausted its supply of oxygen (deoxygenated blood) is transported back to the right side of the heart via the **superior vena cava** (coming from the upper body) and the **inferior vena cava** (from the lower body).

It enters the right atrium and then travels through the **tricuspid valve** to the right ventricle. From here, it leaves the heart via the right and left pulmonary arteries to the corresponding right or left lung.

In the lungs, the pulmonary arteries become smaller arterioles and then even smaller capillaries. The capillaries have walls that are one cell thick; they form a mesh around the lower end of the airways, where there are tiny dilated sacs called alveoli (see Figure 14.3). This is where inhaled oxygen can be transferred across the very thin walls of the airways and surrounding capillaries into the bloodstream. The alveoli are shaped like bunches of grapes to increase the surface area across which the gases can be exchanged, and this makes the process more efficient.

Carbon dioxide (CO_2, the waste gas produced from metabolism in all the organs of the body) is also transferred from the blood back into the airways to be exhaled.

The reoxygenated blood is now transported back through the pulmonary veins to the left atrium. From here, it travels through the **mitral valve** into the left ventricle. This is the largest chamber in the heart, and when it contracts, it squeezes the blood with its vital oxygen out through the aorta.

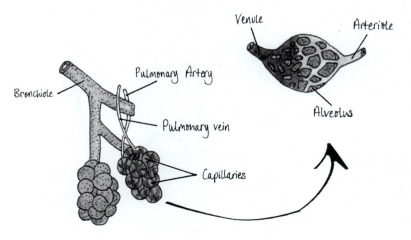

Figure 14.3 Alveolus

The aorta divides into an ascending aorta, sending blood to the upper body, and the descending aorta, sending blood to the lower body.

This vital transport system can only be maintained if the heart beats at an appropriate rate.

WHAT MAKES THE HEART CONTRACT?

The heart is a muscle. Inside the right atrium, there is an area of specialised heart tissue called the sinus node or sino-atrial (SA) node (see Figure 14.2). This node produces an electrical impulse that travels down through the right atrium to another area of specialised tissue called the atrioventricular node. From here, the electrical impulses travel down through the **bundle of His** and spread out around the heart muscle, causing it to contract. When the ventricles contract, the blood is pushed out through the arteries.

These electrical currents spread through the whole body. They can be picked up by applying electrodes to various parts of the body and connecting them to an electrocardiograph (ECG). The ECG is a graphic recording of electrical processes that make the heart muscle contract.

Abnormalities result in changes in the ECG and can help with diagnosis, depending on the extent and position of the changes.

The ECG detects the electrical current flowing through the heart, and depending on the size and state of the heart muscle, it will produce deflections on the ECG monitor.

It also shows the heart rate and rhythm.

PQRST

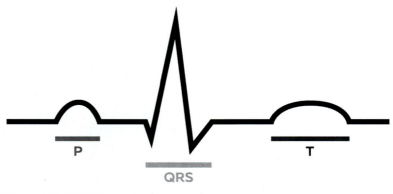

Figure 14.4 PQRST complex

- P represents the electrical activity during contraction of the smaller chambers (atria).
- QRS represents the current that causes contraction of the left and right ventricles. Because the ventricles have a larger muscle mass than the atria, there is a larger deflection on the ECG recording.
- T represents the repolarisation (like a resetting of the spring) of the ventricles. The repolarisation of the atria is hidden in the QRS complex (see Figure 14.4).

HEART DISEASE

Various types of heart disease that affect the heart muscle or interfere with the rate or rhythm may be detected on an ECG.

Ischaemic heart disease

Remember, the heart is a muscle, so it also needs an independent blood supply to obtain its oxygen and nutrients. This is delivered via the right and left coronary arteries.

In heart disease, these arteries may be narrow or blocked by fatty deposits called atheroma. This restricts the flow of blood to the heart muscle (**ischaemia**). The restriction is initially more of a problem when the heart muscle is working hard, as in exercise or exertion. The heart needs more blood for its supply of oxygen and nutrients, and if the blood supply is compromised, the heart muscle will not be able to work properly and will become painful. This is what causes the pain of **angina**, which is typically felt during exertion or stress. The pain will go after rest unless there is a complete blockage or clot. In this case, the pain will not go with rest as the affected muscle is completely deprived of oxygen and it dies (heart attack or **myocardial infarction**; see Figure 14.5). When this happens, the outcome will depend on where the blockage has occurred. If it is at the end of one of the tiny branches of the coronary artery, it may only be experienced as a feeling of indigestion for a while (a silent heart attack), and this may only be detected on a subsequent ECG. If the blockage is further up the coronary artery, it will affect a larger area of heart muscle, and may cause the heart to stop (cardiac arrest), depending on the amount of heart muscle involved.

The pain of angina or a heart attack may be felt in the chest, jaw or left arm. Occasionally, it may be felt in the right arm. This is because of the way in which the nerves are distributed in the chest wall. Other possible symptoms may include a feeling of pressure in the chest, indigestion, nausea, vomiting, sweating, shortness of breath, and feeling dizzy or faint.

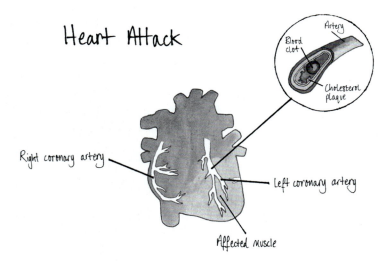

Figure 14.5 Heart attack

The ECG recording may look different in someone who has ischaemic heart disease or who has had a heart attack. This is because the muscle may be damaged, so the flow of electric current through the muscle is altered and the deflections on the recording will be different.

Atrial fibrillation (AF)

This occurs when the sinus node fires erratic impulses, causing the atria to 'fibrillate' or quiver as they beat very rapidly and irregularly. Because the atria are beating so fast (sometimes more than 300bpm), the blood is not pumped through to the ventricles effectively and it may pool in the left atria, where it is then more likely to form clots. If the clots break loose and are pumped around the body, they can then lodge in blood vessels in the brain and cause a stroke, or they may block an artery supplying the heart and cause a heart attack.

The ECG recording will look different in AF. Because the atria are not beating properly, the P wave does not show up clearly on the ECG recording. It may only appear as a fibrillatory line like a series of small bumps. This is very characteristic of AF.

Heart failure

This is when the heart cannot pump the full amount of blood with each heartbeat, and is therefore unable to meet the needs of the body. It is classified as systolic and diastolic failure, and may affect only the right ventricle or the left ventricle, or both

It is commonly caused by heart disease, such as after a heart attack, or may occur because of uncontrolled hypertension. It may also be a complication of AF or valve disease.

It is estimated that over one million people in the UK have heart failure (BHF 2024).

The incidence rises steeply with age and carries a poor prognosis that is worse than most cancers, with a high percentage of patients diagnosed with heart failure dying within a year, usually because by the time it is diagnosed, it is quite advanced. The emphasis should be on diagnosing heart failure early to ensure that the problem can be treated more quickly to prevent early complications (Taylor et al. 2019).

There are many possible symptoms, including shortness of breath, swelling of the feet and legs, a chronic lack of energy, difficulty sleeping due to breathing problems, a swollen or tender abdomen and a loss of appetite, a cough with frothy sputum, increased urination at night, and confusion or an impaired memory.

The ECG recording may show the possible *cause* of heart failure, such as AF or a previous myocardial infarction, and it may demonstrate possible signs of heart failure such as an enlarged left ventricle (left ventricular hypertrophy). It can be useful to signal the need for further investigations, but it cannot provide a definitive diagnosis.

THE 12-LEAD ECG

When detecting any abnormalities in the current flowing through the heart, the ECG can determine *where* the abnormality may be. It does this by viewing the heart from different directions. To record an ECG, there are six chest electrodes and four limb electrodes, but it becomes a little confusing because it is referred to as a 12-lead ECG (see Figure 14.6).

So how does 6 + 4 = a 12-lead ECG?

- A lead is a view of the electrical activity of the heart from a particular angle across the body, obtained by using signals from different combinations of electrodes.
- To obtain a 12-lead ECG, you have one electrode attached to each of the limbs and six electrodes placed on the chest, ten in total, but you get 12 'leads', or pictures from the combinations of different electrodes.
- For the chest, the six leads take their picture (or view) from an electrode each, and are referred to as unipolar (leads V1–V6).

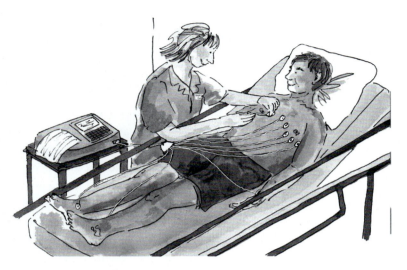

Figure 14.6 HCA performing an ECG

- Three of the limb leads are made up from the signals of two electrodes each, and are referred to as bipolar (leads I–III).
- The other three limb leads are made up from signals of three electrodes each, and are called augmented leads (aVF, aVR, aVL).
- The electrode placed on the right foot serves only as an earth, and does not play a part in the recording.

Some reasons for performing an ECG

- Chest pain? Always make sure you have professional help at hand in case of sudden deterioration in the patient.
- History of chest pain or heart attack.
- Hypertension.
- Palpitations.
- Patient at risk.
- Prior to some drug treatments.
- Shortness of breath.

RECORDING AN ECG: THE PROCEDURE (ADAPTED FROM SCST 2024)

You can download the National Occupational Standard CHS130 *Perform Routine Electrocardiograph Procedures* to use as a checklist for your competencies (Skills for Health 2021).

Preparing the patient

Good preparation is an essential part of the process in the quest for the most accurate ECG recording, as follows.

1 Confirm the patient's identity and make sure this correlates with the name on the computer screen.
2 Explain the process, including what will happen before, during and after the procedure. Ensure that the patient understands and is happy to proceed (obtain informed consent).
3 Consider privacy and comfort in what can be a distressing and embarrassing procedure for some patients. A trained chaperone should be offered according to the local policy.
4 The patient should be in a semi-recumbent position of approximately 45 degrees, and any significant variation from this should be recorded. The limbs should be supported.
5 There should be unrestricted access to the chest, arms and legs. While respecting the cultural sensitivities of the patient, ask them to remove all clothing that may impede access to the electrode positions. Remember to offer a 'dignity blanket' for female patients to minimise embarrassment.
6 Reassure the anxious patient. Anxiety will make the heart beat faster, so the result will not be accurate. Make sure they understand that the ECG is a recording of electrical activity *from* them and is not a current being passed *through* them!
7 If the skin is sweaty or oily, clean it with a mild detergent or alcohol wipe to ensure a good contact. Similarly, if the patient has a lot of chest hair, it is sometimes necessary to shave those areas where the electrodes are to be stuck on. Always use a disposable single-use razor. If **exfoliation** is required, rub the skin lightly with a paper towel, gauze swab or abrasive tape designed for the purpose.
8 Discourage any talking or movement, as this involves the use of other muscles. Make sure the patient's fists are not clenched. All muscles contract because of electrical stimulus, so there is the potential for this to interfere with the recording from the heart.
9 It is important to *place the electrodes consistently and in the recommended positions* to achieve the most accurate recording. Studies have shown that electrodes are frequently placed incorrectly, producing significant diagnostic differences (Kligfield et al. 2007; Kania et al. 2014). Because of this, there are recommended positions

that should be adhered to whenever possible, or – if not possible – then the alternative positions used should be documented. Electrodes on the limbs and chest should be placed as in Table 14.1 (see also Figure 14.7).

Table 14.1 Recommended positions for the electrodes

Electrode	Recommended position
Red	Inside the right wrist
Yellow	Inside the left wrist
Green	Inside the left ankle
Black	Inside the right ankle
V1	Fourth right **intercostal space** at **sternal border**
V2	Fourth left intercostal space at sternal border
V3	Midway between V2 and V4
V4	Fifth left intercostal space in **midclavicular line**
V5	Left **anterior** axillary line at same horizontal level as V4
V6	Left mid-axillary line at same horizontal level as V4

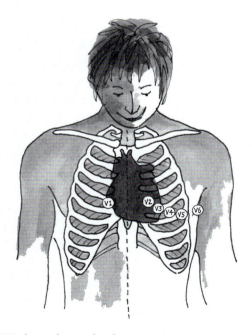

Figure 14.7 ECG electrodes on the chest

Tips for remembering the limb leads

It may be helpful to remember the mnemonic 'ride your green bike' (RYGB) as a memory aid for the sequence of limb electrode colours. The red electrode is applied to the inside of the right wrist, the yellow electrode to the inside of the left wrist, the green electrode to the left foot, and the black electrode to the right foot.

When a patient has a tremor or is an amputee, it may be necessary to position the limb lead on the corresponding shoulder or lower torso. Always document any variation from the regular position.

Tips for placing the chest leads

To identify the fourth intercostal space for the chest leads, it may be helpful to slide a finger from the base of the throat downwards as far as a bony lump (angle of Louis). Then slide the finger to the left or right to identify the second intercostal space. From this position, run your fingers downward across the next rib and the next one. You are now in the fourth intercostal space.

Alternatively, count the dips in between the ribs, starting at the clavicle and working downwards to the fourth dip, but take care not to count the very first small dip between the clavicle and first rib.

Chest leads 3–5 can be placed under or over breast tissue.

10 Once the electrodes have been applied and good contact ensured, press the button to start the machine and record a 12-lead ECG at 25 mm/second with a gain setting of 10 mm/mv. All filters should be off for the first attempt because use of the filter may distort the ECG. The filter setting should only be used if there is interference from other muscle movement, and should be clearly marked on the recording. If the rhythm is irregular, an additional rhythm strip should be recorded, usually on lead II for a minimum of ten seconds. This must be done manually.

11 When the recording is done, ensure correct labelling and show it to the requesting practitioner before the patient leaves the surgery (or proceed according to the local protocol).

12 Scan it immediately on to the computer and make sure the paper recording is stored away from the clinical area to preserve confidentiality.

Other factors to consider

Infection control

Observe correct hand decontamination before and after the procedure, and clean the couch between patients. Dispose of couch roll and disposable razors in line with your local policy.

Health and safety

Make sure the couch is at the correct height. Ideally, couches in the treatment room should be adjustable so that the patient can get on and off safely and the practitioner can attend to the patient without bending. Take care when helping patients on or off the couch.

All electrical equipment should be checked annually and the date recorded on the equipment. It should also be calibrated annually or as recommended by the manufacturer.

Dextrocardia

This is a common form of cardiac malposition where the heart is positioned on the right side rather than the left side. In this case, V1 and V2 can stay in the same position, but V3–V6 should be positioned on the right side of the chest using the same intercostal spacing and anatomical landmarks as previously described.

Now try the following quiz. You can check back in the text for the answers.

HEART AND ECG QUIZ

1. List three reasons why a patient might need to have an ECG.
2. What are the four chambers of the heart called?
3. Which blood vessels carry blood away from the heart?
4. Which vein carries blood back to the heart from the upper body?
5. Where do the pulmonary arteries carry the blood to, and why?
6. Which area of the heart normally produces the electrical impulse that makes the heart muscle contract?
7. How should the patient be positioned to have an ECG?
8. Where would you place the electrode V2?
9. Where would you place the red electrode?
10. How do you get 12 leads (pictures) from ten electrodes?

TIME TO REFLECT

 Using a framework for reflection (see Chapter 2), try reflecting on a consultation when you performed an ECG recording.

How did it go, and what did you learn?

 The ups and downs in life are important to keep us going because a straight line, even in an ECG, means we're not alive!

REFERENCES

BHF (2024) *UK Factsheet*. https://www.bhf.org.uk/-/media/files/for-professionals/research/heart-statistics/bhf-cvd-statistics-uk-factsheet.pdf (accessed September 13, 2024).

Kania, M., Rix, H., Ferenie, M. et al. (2014) The effect of precordial lead displacement on ECG morphology. *Medical & Biological Engineering & Computing* 52(2): 109–119. https://www.ncbi.nlm.nih.gov/pmc/articles/PMC3899452/ (accessed September 13, 2024).

Kligfield, P., Gettes, L., Bailey, J. et al. (2007) Recommendations for the standardisation and interpretation of the electrocardiogram. *Circulation* 115(10): 1306–1324. https://www.ncbi.nlm.nih.gov/pubmed/17322457 (accessed September 13, 2024).

SCST (2024) *Recording a Standard 12-Lead Electrocardiogram*. https://scst.org.uk/wp-content/uploads/2024/09/2024_ECG_Recording_Guidelines_26-09-2024_V5_FINAL.pdf (accessed November 4, 2024).

Skills for Health (2021) *CHS130 Perform Routine Electrocardiograph ECG Procedures*. https://tools.skillsforhealth.org.uk/competence-details/html/4379 (accessed September 13, 2024).

Taylor, C., Ordonez-Mena, J., Roalfe, A.K. et al. (2019) Trends in survival after a diagnosis of heart failure in the UK 2000–2017: Population based cohort study. *BMJ* 364: l223. https://www.bmj.com/content/bmj/364/bmj.l223.full.pdf (accessed September 13, 2024).

Venepuncture and capillary blood testing

Best practice

15

Venepuncture is a task that is often one of the first to be taken on by an HCA, and many will be extremely proficient in the procedure. It is, however, another one of those tasks which is so essential to get right to achieve the best and most accurate sample possible. This may sound obvious, but it is surprising how many errors 'competent' phlebotomists can make that can have significant implications for the patient. This chapter will provide some of the necessary underpinning knowledge in the physiological process and will outline the correct procedure to achieve accurate sampling.

Before you consider performing venepuncture, make sure you are up to date with your hepatitis B protection.

THE CLOTTING PROCESS IN VENEPUNCTURE

When a hole is made in the vein by a needle, platelets (small fragments of blood cells) become sticky and clump around the injury. Activated platelets and injured tissue produce chemicals that react with clotting factors in the blood. These clotting factors are known by the Roman numerals I–XIII. Factor I (fibrinogen) is converted into thin strands of solid protein called fibrin. These strands trap the platelets and blood cells to form a solid clot or plug. This process may take several hours, so it is important to remind the patient not to do anything after the procedure that may interfere with this, or they risk further bleeding and subsequent bruising.

Factors that may interfere with the clotting process

- Abnormal liver function (the liver produces the clotting factors).
- Vitamin K levels (because factors II, VII, IX and X are dependent on Vitamin K).
- Clotting disorders such as **haemophilia**.

DOI: 10.4324/9781003460381-19

- **Anticoagulants** such as aspirin, warfarin and heparin.
- **Hypercoaguability** disorders (whereby the blood clots too easily).
- Low platelet counts such as in **immunosuppression** or **leukaemia**.
- Platelet function disorders.
- Heavy lifting or excessive movement within two hours of venepuncture.

ORDER OF DRAW

Blood samples should be drawn in the correct order to avoid **cross-contamination** of additives between tubes (Bazzano et al. 2021).

Check with your local laboratory for current guidelines regarding which colour sample bottles to use for which test and the order of draw. As a general rule, blood glucose samples should be taken last in the order of draw as these bottles contain an **enzyme** that may adversely affect other tests if there is any cross-contamination.

FACTORS AFFECTING THE QUALITY OF THE SAMPLE

There are some factors that may affect the results of a blood sample that the blood-taker cannot do anything about, such as the patient's age, gender, race, pregnancy and so on. There are other factors that may affect the quality that will depend very much on the competence of the blood-taker.

When a blood sample is analysed in the laboratory, the levels of various substances that are present in the fluid part of the blood are measured. *Haemolysis* is the term used to describe the damage of red blood cells, which results in leakage of their contents into the blood serum. When a blood sample is haemolysed, the test may give a false high reading for substances such as potassium. This is because most of the potassium in the body is intracellular (contained within the cells). When the cell is damaged, the potassium leaks out into the serum, so the blood sample will give a false high reading. Potassium is very important for muscle contraction, particularly of the heart muscle, so patients who have a high potassium level will always need to be retested promptly.

ACTIVITY

List as many things as you can think of that may cause damage to the blood cells during and after venepuncture, or that may give inaccurate results for other reasons.

How could this affect patient care?

Check your answers in Box 15.1.

A BIT ABOUT TOURNIQUETS

Many areas now recommend the use of single-use tourniquets, but if these are not available, then you should use tourniquets with a quick and slow release mechanism. Position the tourniquet 10 cm (a hand width) above the intended puncture site. It should be loosened or removed when the first tube starts to fill, and never left on for longer than is necessary. **Always** remove the tourniquet before removing the needle from the vein.

If the vein is clearly visible and **palpable**, consider taking the blood *without* using a tourniquet. Prolonged use may be uncomfortable and can cause haemolysis, adversely affecting the quality of the sample.

Research has identified contamination of reusable tourniquets most commonly with *Staphylococcus* (Szymczyk et al. 2023). It is possible, of course, that this contamination comes from the blood takers hands after inadequate hand-washing between patients, rather than from the patient.

There is an ongoing debate about the need for disposable tourniquets. The problem with these is that many of them do not incorporate a slow release mechanism, so they are either on or off. There is therefore no way to retighten the tourniquet easily if the blood flow stops. Furthermore, disposable tourniquets are seen as expensive and not environmentally friendly. Each reusable tourniquet can be reused for two years or 10,000 uses. This avoids plastic waste equivalent to 2.3tonnes of CO_2 (NHS Supply Chain 2023).

If reusable tourniquets are used, then consider washing them at the end of every session and never use them if they are visibly contaminated. You must always use the type of tourniquet stated in your local policy.

VENEPUNCTURE: THE PROCEDURE

You can download the National Occupational Standard CHS 132 *Obtain Venous Blood Samples* to use as a checklist for your competencies (Skills for Health 2021a).

1 Identify the patient by asking them to say their name and address and date of birth (you must have at least three points of reference).
2 Obtain informed verbal consent before proceeding. Make sure the patient understands why they are having their blood taken and what the possible risks of the procedure are, including possible bruising.
3 Check the history. Has the patient had any previous problems with the procedure or any surgery to one side where use of the opposite

arm may be advised (e.g. **lymph node clearance**)? Have they fasted if necessary?

4   Position the patient appropriately. Always lie them down if they have fainted before or if they are unsure. The chair should ideally be designed for the purpose, but failing this, it should – as a minimum requirement – have arms to prevent the patient falling to the side.

5   Decontaminate your hands and put on gloves (NHS England 2022 updated 2024).

6   Prepare the equipment:

- Blood collection bottles according to the tests to be collected (charts with blood bottle colours are available from all hospital pathology laboratories). Always put a spare set of bottles on the tray in case there are problems obtaining the blood. Check that bottles are in date.
- Two needles (one spare): 20-, 21- and 22-gauge needles are all suitable.
- Cotton wool ball.
- Alcohol wipe.
- Tourniquet.
- Plaster or **hypoallergenic** tape.
- Sharps box.
- Bottle holder (if using the vacuette system).

7   Identify the best arm and expose the antecubital fossa (i.e. inside the elbow; see Figure 15.1). Avoid using the weak or paralysed arm if the patient has had a stroke. Any tight clothing should be removed. Support the patient's arm on a pad and advise the patient to keep the arm straight throughout the procedure. Look for the most visible and palpable, or 'bouncy', vein. The median cubital vein is

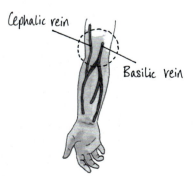

Figure 15.1 Antecubital fossa

usually the easiest to puncture. The basilic vein may be used, but as it usually runs above the brachial artery and nerve there is a greater risk of an arterial stab or nerve damage, so it is best avoided if possible. Where there isn't a good visible vein, apply the tourniquet and take time to carefully palpate the area to identify the best vein. Time taken at this stage is time well spent! Try to avoid choosing a site where the veins are diverging, as there is more risk of a bruise forming. Loosen the tourniquet once the vein is located.

8 Now clean the area using an alcohol wipe, working with a firm downward and outward motion across the whole area for 30 seconds (WHO 2010). In some areas, this step is omitted from the policy, as there is no good evidence to support the cleansing of skin prior to the procedure. Check your local policy and if the skin is visibly dirty, it should be washed with soap and water.
9 Prepare the equipment.
10 Retighten the tourniquet if being used and if necessary.

Vacuette system (used in most areas in England and Wales)

- Attach the needle to the holder (vacuette).
- Drop the sheath off the needle at 90 degrees to avoid any spur on the needle that might occur when the sheath is pulled off horizontally.
- Warn the patient to expect a sharp scratch. Insert the needle, **bevel** upwards, into the vein at a 30-degree angle to about half the length of the needle.

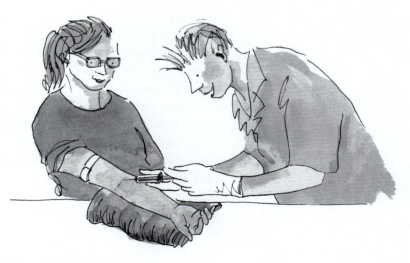

Figure 15.2 HCA taking blood

- Push on the first bottle (observing the order of draw) while firmly anchoring the holder so that the needle doesn't move in the vein.
- When the blood starts to flow, loosen the tourniquet if it has been tightened. Allow the blood to finish filling the tube completely before gently removing and inverting the tube twice.
- Apply the next bottle and repeat the procedure.

Monovette system (used in some areas)

- Attach the needle to the first bottle (observing the order of draw) and twist to lock. Drop the sheath off the needle at 90 degrees to avoid any spur on the needle that might occur if the sheath is pulled off horizontally.
- Warn the patient to expect a sharp scratch.
- Insert the needle, bevel upwards, into the vein at a 30-degree angle to about half the length of the needle.
- Pull out the plunger of the bottle until it clicks, taking care not to move the needle in the vein.
- When the blood starts to flow, loosen the tourniquet if it has been tightened.
- Allow the bottle to finish filling the tube completely before removing and inverting twice.
- Attach the next bottle and repeat. Second and subsequent bottles can be prepared by pulling out the plunger until it clicks and then snapping it off.

Finishing up:

1 *Before* taking the needle out, remember to remove the tourniquet.
2 Remove the needle and then apply the cotton wool, advising the patient to press firmly for a few minutes (they may need to press for longer if on anticoagulant therapy).
3 Pick up all the bottles and invert fully again a further four times (so six in total). Check your laboratory chart, as many will now specify how many times each bottle should be inverted.
4 Label the bottles, checking details with the patient, and put into the pathology bag/form.
5 Apply an appropriate dressing to the venepuncture site (always check for allergies first).
6 Dispose of sharps and equipment immediately, according to local policy.

7 Remove gloves and decontaminate hands.

8 Advise the patient about aftercare and follow-up.

9 Document the procedure. Include consent obtained, which blood tests were taken, who the requesting practitioner was, which arm was used and any problems that were encountered.

TROUBLESHOOTING

What will you do if any of the following occur?

- *The patient faints during the procedure.* This depends on if they are safe or not. If they are lying down and quite safe, continue with the procedure. It is much better to do this than to have to go through the whole procedure again if it makes them faint! If they are not safe, take off the tourniquet and remove the needle. Advise the patient to lean forward with their head down or to lie down. Apply a dressing to the venepuncture site. Support the patient gently to the floor if necessary and elevate the legs. Recovery from a simple faint is usually quite quick, but they may need a glass of water and observation for a short while. If the blood has not been taken at this stage, refer them to a registered practitioner for further tests. Always have the patient checked over by a registered practitioner before they leave the surgery if they have been unwell.

- *An artery is punctured instead of a vein.* This is an uncommon event but can happen, especially when choosing a vein on the inner edge of the antecubital fossa. This is where the brachial artery is usually situated, but it is deeper and can be distinguished from a vein because the artery will have a pulse and will not 'plump up' when the tourniquet is applied. Blood from an artery will pump into the collection bottle in spurts and will be a brighter red colour than that from a vein. If this happens, take the tourniquet off and remove the needle. You should apply pressure for a minimum of five minutes and apply a pressure dressing when bleeding has stopped. Ask a registered practitioner to assess the patient before attempting venepuncture again or before the patient leaves the surgery.

- *The vein 'collapses'.* This usually means that the vacuum has sucked the wall of the vein on to the needle and stopped the flow of blood. This can sometimes be overcome by taking the bottle off and then reapplying or by gently tilting the needle in the vein.

- *There is no blood flow.* The needle may have gone through the vein or missed it completely. Gently and very slowly withdraw or manoeuvre the needle until the blood starts to flow. If there is still no success, slowly take the needle out, checking all the time for any indication of blood flow. Repeat the procedure with a fresh needle and bottle. Do not make more than two attempts on each arm.

AN OVERVIEW OF SOME COMMON BLOOD TESTS

Full blood count (FBC)

This tells us how many red blood cells, white blood cells and platelets there are. It also identifies the different types of white blood cells. The shape and size of the cells can be determined. *Red blood cells* carry essential oxygen attached to **haemoglobin**. Because of this, a reduction in the number of red blood cells or a problem with them can result in a shortage of oxygen in the body. *White blood cells* (made up of neutrophils, lymphocytes, monocytes, basophils and eosinophils) fight different types of infection and are essential in the immune system. *Platelets* are small fragments of cells that are important in the clotting process.

The FBC is a **haematological test**, and may be done for several reasons, including the following:

- hypertension (because too many red blood cells can make the blood thicker and increase the blood pressure);
- heart disease;
- COPD;
- diabetes;
- any prolonged or recurrent infection;
- cancer – undergoing chemotherapy;
- inflammatory diseases requiring disease-modifying antirheumatic drugs (DMARDs), such as methotrexate; and
- anaemia.

Erythrocyte sedimentation rate (ESR)

Inflammatory processes affect the red blood cells and prolong the time it takes to spin them down in a centrifuge. The **erythrocyte** sedimentation rate (ESR) can indicate if there is any inflammation going on in the body. It will also be influenced by age and gender.

The ESR should be measured within two hours of the blood being taken to achieve the most accurate result.

Kidney or renal function tests (RFTs), also referred to as urea and electrolytes (U&Es)

The kidneys are two small organs positioned either side of the back in the left and right loin. They are essential organs and act as filters for the blood, sieving out waste products and excreting them in the urine. When the kidneys are not functioning properly, toxic waste products can build up in the blood and interfere with the normal functioning of the body.

Kidney function tests are performed to measure the levels of urea, creatinine and electrolytes, including sodium, potassium, chloride and bicarbonate. Some of the reasons for checking kidney function include:

- kidney disease;
- hypertension;
- diabetes; and
- when the patient is taking specific medications such as some antihypertensives.

The kidney function test will also identify the glomerular filtration rate (GFR), which indicates the rate at which the kidney is filtering the blood, and can therefore give information about the health and efficiency of the kidney.

Liver function tests (LFTs)

The liver is a vital organ in the right upper part of the abdomen. It has several essential functions:

- storage of glycogen (made from sugars – this is the fuel for the body);
- metabolising (breaking down) fats and proteins from food;
- processing and metabolising many toxins and drugs;
- production of vitamin K and other chemicals needed to help the blood clot; and
- production of bile (stored in the gall bladder), which is necessary for digesting fats.

LFTs measure the levels of liver enzymes – such as alkaline phosphatase (ALP), alanine transaminase (ALT) and aspartate aminotransferase (AST) – and abnormal levels may indicate liver disease. LFTs also measure albumin (the main protein produced by the liver), total protein and bilirubin, which gives the bile its green-yellow colour and may make the patient look yellow (jaundiced) when there are high levels in the blood.

Another test of the liver that may be done if requested is the gamma-glutamyl transferase (GGT). High levels may indicate alcohol abuse as well as other types of liver disease.

Some reasons for checking liver function are:

- to help diagnose and monitor liver disease; and
- as a precaution after starting some drugs, such as **statins**, to check that they are not causing liver damage.

Calcium

Calcium is an essential mineral, and about 99% is found in the bones and teeth, with the rest found in the blood and soft tissues. It is vital for healthy bones and teeth, and to help with muscle contractions, blood clotting and nerve function.

Calcium levels may be checked in patients with:

- kidney stones;
- bone disease;
- neurological (nerve) disease;
- kidney disease;
- symptoms of high calcium (e.g. fatigue, weakness, **anorexia**, vomiting, constipation, thirst, urinary frequency);
- symptoms of low calcium (e.g. abdominal cramps, muscle cramps, tingling fingers); and
- other diseases that may be associated with abnormal calcium levels, such as thyroid disease, cancer, malnutrition and intestinal disease.

> Some literature advises against the use of the tourniquet when checking calcium levels, as it has been suggested that prolonged use of the tourniquet gives a falsely high reading. However, this is controversial and will depend on laboratory testing methods. Check with your local laboratory.

Blood glucose

Diabetes is a disease by which the body either does not produce any insulin, or it may produce some but the body is resistant to it. Insulin is a chemical that is produced by the pancreas, and it is essential to enable glucose circulating in the blood to enter the cells of the body for them to function properly. When the blood glucose cannot enter the cells, the levels in the blood will rise, and subsequent high levels over time can cause many problems, such as heart disease and strokes, eye damage, kidney damage, and damage to the nerves, causing numbness or pain in the feet and hands.

Diabetes can be diagnosed by measuring blood glucose levels, but it is now usually diagnosed by measuring the glycated or glycosylated haemoglobin (HbA1C).

A *random blood glucose level* of 11.1 mmol/L or more indicates diabetes. This will usually be confirmed with a fasting test.

A *fasting blood glucose level* of 7.0 mmol/L or more indicates diabetes but will usually be repeated to confirm the diagnosis.

When the levels are on the borderline and the diagnosis is in doubt, the patient will sometimes be referred for an oral glucose tolerance test. For this test, the patient must fast overnight and then have a blood sample taken. They are then given a glucose drink. A blood sample taken again two hours later showing a glucose level of greater than 11 mmol/L indicates that the body is unable to deal efficiently with the glucose and confirms the diagnosis of diabetes. This test is also done routinely in pregnancy when the expectant mother is larger than expected, as a large baby can sometimes occur when the mother has gestational diabetes.

HbA1C

When there is an excess of glucose in the blood system, it will attach freely to haemoglobin in the red blood cells. Red blood cells live for about 120 days, so measuring the haemoglobin that has glucose attached to it (glycated haemoglobin) indicates the levels of circulating glucose in the bloodstream over the past three to four months. It is much more useful to determine the overall diabetic control, as a fasting glucose level will only indicate the immediate glucose level. The HbA1C is now also used to diagnose diabetes, and a level of 6.5% or greater is a positive result.

Thyroid function tests

The thyroid gland is situated in the neck, and it produces hormones that increase the body's metabolic rate and help to control the level of calcium in the blood.

Thyroid function tests are done to diagnose thyroid disorders and to monitor people who have an underactive thyroid gland (hypothyroidism) and who take thyroid replacement medication (thyroxine). They are also done to monitor people who have an overactive thyroid (hyperthyroidism) and who take other types of drugs to counter the effects of this.

Newborn babies are checked for inherited thyroid problems.

The first test will usually be for the thyroid-stimulating hormone (TSH), which is responsible for stimulating the gland to produce the hormones T4 and T3. Levels of these hormones will be checked if the TSH levels are abnormal.

Lipid profile test

Lipid is basically fat, and it is stored in the body as a source of energy. A lipid profile includes measurements of cholesterol, triglycerides, low-density **lipoprotein** (LDL) and high-density lipoprotein (HDL).

- *Cholesterol* is a fat made in the liver from fats in the food we eat. We all need some cholesterol, as it forms an important component of the cell walls in our body. It is carried in the bloodstream by the lipoproteins HDL and LDL.
- *HDL* is the transporter of 'good cholesterol', and higher levels are associated with reduced fatty deposits in the arteries (atheroma).
- *LDL* is the transporter of 'bad cholesterol', and it is the LDL that is implicated in the formation of atheroma.
- *Triglycerides* are the end product of the metabolism of the bulky fats present in food. Triglycerides are stored in adipose (fat) cells to be used as energy if food is unavailable.

Hyperlipidaemia can occur in people who have an unhealthy diet but can also be inherited. It may be secondary to other conditions, such as diabetes, thyroid disease and some liver and kidney disorders. It is an important risk factor for heart disease and strokes.

Historically, diagnosis has been made after a fasting blood test (fasting for 12 hours with only water to drink), but this is no longer considered appropriate or necessary (NICE 2023).

Occasionally, a doctor may still order a fasting test of triglycerides if non-fasting values have been significantly elevated because they can be affected for several hours by a high-fat meal.

High LDL levels are associated with a higher risk of heart disease, and should be less than 3.0 mmol/L. However, the ratio of total cholesterol to HDL (TC:HDL ratio) is also an important indicator, and should be 4.5 mmol/L or less.

International normalised ratio (INR)

This is a measure of how much longer it takes the blood to clot than normal, so if the INR is measured as 2.0, the blood is taking twice as long as normal to clot. For most of us, assuming we are not taking any anticoagulant medication, our INR would be 1.0. The INR is a test used most commonly for patients who are taking warfarin.

Warfarin blocks the effects of vitamin K and depletes the clotting factors in the body, so it inhibits the formation of clots. This is useful in patients with certain types of medical conditions, such as:

- atrial fibrillation;
- **deep-vein thrombosis (DVT)** or **pulmonary embolism**; and
- mechanical heart valves or heart valve disease.

Each patient who takes warfarin will need an individualised, specific dose that is titrated according to the INR result. For this reason, it is essential to make sure you achieve a good-quality sample so that the patient receives an appropriate therapeutic dose. An overdose of warfarin can have catastrophic effects, resulting in the patient bleeding to death, and conversely – if the warfarin dose is too low for that patient – they are at greater risk of complications, including a stroke.

Blood sample bottles for INR testing contain heparin, which stops the blood from clotting so it can be tested accurately.

This principle applies to other blood tests, as well – additives in the various blood sample tubes are measured for a specific amount of blood.

> Always make sure that the blood sample bottle is filled to the mark on the tube. If the ratio of blood in the tube is not enough for the heparin additive in the tube, the INR will be recorded as much higher than it is. If you have difficulty 'bleeding' a patient, always document this on the form so that the laboratory staff can make allowances for this.

CAPILLARY BLOOD TESTING

This is useful when only a very small amount of blood is needed or when venepuncture is difficult. It is a convenient way of monitoring blood glucose, INR and cholesterol levels.

It is not without potential pitfalls, however, and the person performing the test must ensure that it is done correctly to provide as accurate a result as possible.

Capillary blood testing: the procedure

You can download the National Occupational Standard CHS 131 *Obtain and Test Capillary Blood Samples* to use as a checklist for your competencies (Skills for Health 2021b).

1 Confirm the identity of the patient.
2 Obtain verbal informed consent.
3 Decontaminate your hands, put on your gloves and prepare the necessary equipment:

- glucose meter;
- cotton wool or gauze;

Essential Knowledge and Skills for Healthcare Assistants

- appropriate test strip (check that they are in date);
- control solution;
- appropriate device for puncturing the skin;
- clean tray to hold the equipment; and
- sharps box.

4 Make sure the patient's hands are clean, warm and dry before starting.

5 Remove the strip from the foil and insert into the meter with the three black lines at the end of the strip in the meter. The meter will turn on. This will vary according to the device used. Check the manufacturer's instructions if you are unsure.

6 Check that the lot number matches the strip being used (if necessary).

7 Always use a fresh disposable lancet for each patient.

8 Select an appropriate area for puncture.

9 Use the middle, ring or little finger. Puncture the sides of the finger, parallel to the side edges of the nail. Try not to use the tip or pad of the finger because there are more nerve endings there and it will hurt more.

10 If performing the test for blood glucose, wipe away the first drop of blood and discard. Do not do this if checking the INR.

11 Squeeze gently until a rounded bead of blood is obtained. There must be sufficient blood for the meter to function accurately. Do not squeeze the finger too hard. The sample should flow freely from the puncture site. Compress the area, then release for a few seconds and repeat. Take your time! If the flow is too slow, you will need to apply a second puncture.

12 Touch the drop of blood to the white area at the end of the strip until the meter begins the test. Do not remove the test strip or disturb it during the countdown.

Finishing up:

13 Once the sample has been obtained, ask the patient to apply pressure to the site with gauze and maintain pressure until the bleeding has stopped.

14 Dispose of all contaminated items in an approved container.

15 Remove your gloves and decontaminate your hands.

16 Document the result immediately and refer to the doctor or nurse as necessary.

17 Ensure the meter is checked regularly with the local internal quality control tests and external quality control tests (contact your local laboratory for more information).

Perform an internal quality control test:

- daily on meters in use;
- weekly if meters not used often;
- whenever results seem odd; and
- to make sure the meter and strips are working properly.

Do not use the quality control solution if the expiry date has passed. Common sources of error:

- not puncturing the skin deeply enough;
- not wiping away the first drop of blood (for testing glucose levels);
- squeezing too hard or milking the finger excessively;
- using test strips that are past their expiry date; and
- using test strips that have been stored incorrectly and that are damp or damaged.

Accuracy can also be affected by:

- poor peripheral circulation (i.e. poor blood flow to the fingers);
- dehydration;
- hypotension;
- renal dialysis; and
- very high cholesterol levels greater than 13 mmol/L.

Now try the following quiz. You can check back in the text for the answers.

VENEPUNCTURE QUIZ

1. List two factors that might interfere with the clotting process.
2. Which blood bottle should be left until last in the order of draw?
3. What is haemolysis?
4. Assuming you have needed to use a tourniquet, when should you loosen it?
5. When should the tourniquet be removed completely?
6. What will you do if you puncture an artery in error?
7. How many points of reference do you need for labelling the bottles and form?
8. Why do we need red blood cells?
9. List two reasons why a patient may have a kidney function test.
10. Why is it important to fill the blood bottle to the correct level?

Box 15.1 Poor practice in venepuncture: answers to activity

> Poor practice in venepuncture that may give inaccurate results:
>
> - Using needles that are too small or too big.
> - Prolonged use of the tourniquet.
> - Delays in transit time after sampling.
> - Samples stored at the wrong temperature (i.e. in an area that is too warm or too cold). Ideally, samples should be stored in a cool box.
> - Using a thin or 'thready' vein.
> - Taking blood from a bruised area.
> - Not allowing antiseptic skin cleanser to dry.
> - Mixing samples incorrectly or not at all.
> - Bending needles.
> - Filling sample bottles from a syringe and needle.
> - Under-filling the sample.
> - Labelling the sample incorrectly.
>
> Patient care may be compromised, as inaccurate or haemolysed results may result in inappropriate or delayed treatment. Repeat testing is uncomfortable and time-consuming for patients and staff, and is also costly.

TIME TO REFLECT

Using a framework for reflection (see Chapter 2), try reflecting on a consultation when you took blood from a patient.

How did it go, and what did you learn?

You know you're a phlebotomist when you recognise their median antecubital vein rather than the patient's face!

REFERENCES

Bazzano, G., Galazzi, A., Giusti, G.D. et al. (2021) The order of draw during blood collection: A systematic literature review. *International Journal of Environmental Research and Public Health* 18(4): 1568.

https://www.ncbi.nlm.nih.gov/pmc/articles/PMC7915193 (accessed September 13, 2024).

NHS England (2022 updated 2024) *National Infection Prevention and Control Manual (NIPCM) for England*. https://www.england.nhs.uk/national-infection-prevention-and-control-manual-nipcm-for-england (accessed September 18, 2024).

NHS Supply Chain (2023) *Sustainable Reusable Tourniquet Provides Significant Waste Reduction Opportunities for Mid Yorkshire NHS Hospitals Trust*. https://www.supplychain.nhs.uk/news-article/sustainable-reusable-tourniquet-alternative-provides-significant-waste-reduction-opportunities-for-mid-yorkshire-nhs-hospitals-trust (accessed September 18, 2024).

NICE (2023) *Cardiovascular Disease: Risk Assessment and Reduction, Including Lipid Modification*. https://www.nice.org.uk/guidance/ng238/chapter/recommendations#full-lipid-profile (accessed September 18, 2024).

Skills for Health (2021a) *CHS132 Obtain Venous Blood Samples*. https://tools.skillsforhealth.org.uk/competence-details/html/4381 (accessed September 18, 2024).

Skills for Health (2021b) *CHS131 Obtain and Test Capillary Blood Samples*. https://tools.skillsforhealth.org.uk/competence-details/html/4380 (accessed September 18, 2024).

Szymczyk, J., Mansson, M., and Mędrzycka-Dąbrowska, W. (2023) Reusable tourniquets for blood sampling as a source of multi-resistant organisms: A systematic review. *Infectious Diseases: Epidemiology and Prevention* 11: 1258692. https://www.frontiersin.org/journals/public-health/articles/10.3389/fpubh.2023.1258692/full (accessed September 13, 2024)

World Health Organisation [WHO] (2010) *WHO Guidelines on Drawing Blood: Best Practices in Phlebotomy*. https://www.who.int/publications/i/item/9789241599221 (accessed September 18, 2024).

16

Kidney function and urine
Performing accurate urinalysis

Why write a chapter on urinalysis? Surely it just involves dipping a test strip into a pot of urine and reading the result? What could be difficult about that? Of course, there is much more to it as an important diagnostic tool that is all too often very badly performed, resulting in inadequate or inaccurate information and a potentially incorrect diagnosis. As with any other task the HCA performs, it is always easier to perform it well and accurately if there is an understanding of what is being tested for and why.

Urine has historically been used for many different things, and it has had many magical qualities attributed to it. Some tribes in Siberia drink the urine of people who have eaten magic mushrooms in the belief that this will help them communicate with the spirits. Ancient Romans used urine to bleach clothes. It has been used as an antiseptic and as a teeth whitener, and is thought by many different cultures to cure any number of ailments, from acne, warts, hair loss, wrinkles and gastric upset, to name but a few!

Most importantly, though, is the fact that urine testing can tell us a great deal about a person's general health.

WHAT DO THE KIDNEYS DO?

We have two kidneys, both weighing about 160g and measuring 10–15 cm long. They filter the toxins and waste products from the blood, and these are then excreted in the urine.

Each kidney contains approximately two million microscopic sieves or filtering systems called nephrons, which consist of networks of capillaries called glomeruli, where the first phase of filtration occurs. The Bowman's capsule surrounds each glomerulus and is connected to a long tube or 'tubule'. The kidney receives about 1 litre of blood every minute. This blood is filtered through the nephrons and the resulting fluid is sent through the long tubule, where most of the water; essential salts, such as

DOI: 10.4324/9781003460381-20

potassium and sodium; and other substances such as glucose, amino acids and vitamins are reabsorbed back into the bloodstream. The remaining water, urea and other waste substances make up the urine, and this is passed down the ureter to the bladder. Urine is normally made up of 5% salts and ammonia and 95% water.

Approximately 2 litres of urine are produced in 24 hours, but this can vary greatly, and depends on factors such as fluid intake, sweating and general health.

The kidneys are essential for maintaining homeostasis – the normal balance of fluids and salts or electrolytes upon which the proper functioning of the body depends.

The kidneys also secrete some essential hormones such as erythropoietin, which is needed to make red blood cells. For this reason, patients with kidney failure may become anaemic (lacking in oxygen) if they fail to produce enough of this hormone, and therefore lack red blood cells to carry the oxygen.

The nephrons are very delicate structures and easily damaged, especially when pressures are increased, such as in hypertension, or when the renal artery supplying the kidney with blood is narrowed (**renal artery stenosis**). When they are damaged, the sieves or filters become leaky, and larger molecules such as proteins (not normally seen in urine) may become detectable.

WHAT CAN URINE TESTING TELL US?

Look at it

Normal urine is straw coloured and transparent. So, to begin with, have a good look at it and assess if the sample looks normal.

Is it dark or pale? If it is very pale, it indicates a good level of hydration. If very dark, it may indicate **dehydration**.

What colour is it? The colour of the urine can also be altered by medication, foodstuff and disease. Red or pink urine may indicate blood, but may also be caused by eating beetroot! Bright yellow urine can be caused by some vitamins and other medications. Brown urine may indicate the presence of bilirubin if, for example, there is gall bladder disease, but it may also be caused by iron supplements. **Turbid** or cloudy urine may indicate infection. Frothy urine can be due to the presence of glucose or protein.

So, before you have even opened the urine bottle, you may already have some idea of the health, hydration or even diet of the patient.

Smell it

Once you've opened the urine bottle, notice if there is any offensive smell.

A faecal smell could mean that there is a **fistula**, or direct connection between the bowel and bladder where faeces is able to contaminate the urine. A fruity, sweet smell could be significant in a diabetic patient who may have **ketoacidosis**. If the urine smells of asparagus, it is probably because the patient has been eating asparagus! An unpleasant strong smell of ammonia could be due to a bacterial infection.

Dip it

The presence of various substances in the urine that can be detected on the dip test can be very useful to the clinician in making a diagnosis.

Protein should not normally be present in any significant amount, and anything greater than a trace could be significant, so you must take care to observe the colour on the dip test carefully and record the result as accurately as possible. An early morning sample is the best when testing for protein.

Protein may be present in:

- hypertension;
- kidney disease;
- infection;
- inflammation and malignancy;
- diabetes;
- pregnancy – indicating possible **pre-eclampsia**, which is a medical emergency;
- pyrexia;
- dehydration;
- vigorous exercise; and
- 'orthostatic proteinuria', which is usually harmless, and can sometimes be seen in children later in the day.

Blood is not normally present (**haematuria**). Take care when reading the test strip that you allow long enough for the reaction on the strip to occur. For blood, this can take up to two minutes.

Blood may be present in:

- infection;
- trauma or injury to the urinary tract or kidneys;
- kidney stones; and
- malignancy.

It may also be present:

- if the patient is menstruating;
- after vigorous exercise;
- after smoking or toxic chemical exposure; and
- with no known cause – but it should always be reported and investigated.

Ketones are produced by the breakdown of fatty acids.

Ketones may be present in:

- uncontrolled diabetes – so the nurse or doctor should always be informed;
- anorexia or starvation;
- diarrhoea and vomiting;
- pregnancy;
- eclampsia; and
- alcoholism.

Nitrites can be caused by the reaction of some bacteria on urinary nitrates. The pink colour must be uniform to indicate a positive result.

Nitrites may be present when there is infection. However, the test is highly sensitive to air exposure, and will commonly give a false positive result, so some laboratories no longer consider it relevant when deciding if further culture and sensitivity testing is required.

Leucocytes are white blood cells that are usually produced in response to infection.

Leucocytes may be present when there is infection or inflammation in the **genitourinary tract**. There may be false positive results if the test is contaminated by vaginal discharge.

Specific gravity (SG) is often overlooked as a useful test, but can demonstrate the concentration of solutes in the urine.

A low SG might indicate:

- excessive fluid intake;
- renal failure;
- **pyelonephritis**; and
- diabetes insipidus (this is a condition where there is a problem with the adrenal glands, resulting in an inability to control the fluid balance – it is not to be confused with diabetes mellitus).

A high SG shows that the urine is very concentrated with a high level of solutes, and could occur in:

- dehydration;
- renal artery stenosis;
- heart failure; and
- liver failure.

The pH of the urine stands for the 'potential of hydrogen', and demonstrates the concentration of hydrogen ions. This determines whether the urine is alkaline or acidic. Tap water and normal urine will usually be neutral, with a pH of approximately 7.

A pH lower than 7 (acidic urine) may be found:

- in acute starvation;
- in diabetic ketoacidosis;
- when potassium levels are low; and
- when the diet is very acidic.

A pH higher than 7 (alkaline urine) may be found:

- when potassium levels are high; and
- in a vegetarian diet.

Bilirubin is a by-product of the breakdown of red blood cells, and it is normally excreted in the bile. It may be present in urine in liver disease or obstruction of the gall bladder.

URINALYSIS: THE PROCEDURE

You can download the National Occupational Standard HCHS17 *Obtain Specimens from Individuals* to use as a checklist for your competencies (Skills for Health 2010).

1 Always wear gloves.
2 Consider eye protection.
3 Check the expiry date on strips.
4 Immerse the test strip completely in the urine.
5 After dipping in urine, remove any excess urine by tapping the test strip gently on the top of the bottle.
6 Lay the test strip flat on a dry surface.
7 Always check the time and be patient. Some reactions can take up to two minutes. If you do not observe this simple rule, you may miss potentially important results.

Essential Knowledge and Skills for Healthcare Assistants

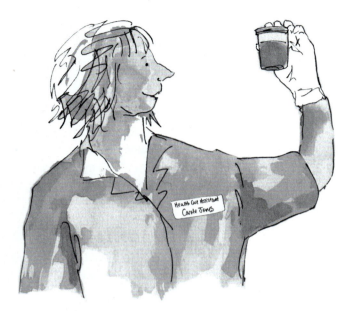

Figure 16.1 HCA testing urine

8   Do not discard urine until you are sure it will not be needed again.
9   Follow infection control procedures and wash your hands thoroughly after removing gloves.
10 Document results accurately.
11 Inform requesting clinician as necessary.

Now try the following quiz. You can check back in the text for the answers.

URINALYSIS QUIZ

1 What do the kidneys do?
2 What factors might influence the amount of urine produced?
3 What does homeostasis mean?
4 What can affect the colour of urine?
5 What is the significance of pale or dark urine?
6 What could cloudy urine indicate?
7 List two conditions that may cause proteinuria.
8 List two conditions that may cause haematuria.
9 Why should you report ketones in the urine?
10 How long should you wait before reading the test strip?

TIME TO REFLECT

 Using a framework for reflection (see Chapter 2), try reflecting on an episode when you performed a urine dip test.

How did it go, and what did you learn?

 Meaning of urine = opposite of 'you're out'!

REFERENCE

Skills for Health (2010) *HCS17 Obtain Specimens from Individuals for Laboratory Investigation.* https://tools.skillsforhealth.org.uk/competence-details/html/2877 (accessed September 18, 2024).

Section IV
More advanced skills

Chapter 17	Examining the feet of people with diabetes	177
Chapter 18	The skin and the healing process: basic wound care	193
Chapter 19	Understanding lung function and disease: performing accurate lung function testing	209
Chapter 20	Administering immunisations	223
Chapter 21	Ear irrigation	253

Examining the feet of people with diabetes

Examining people's feet may not sound like a very pleasant job, but for people who have diabetes, it is vital that their feet are checked regularly. This can be a very suitable role for the HCA or AP who has completed appropriate training. The examination may be performed by the HCA in conjunction with other tests such as BMI, BP and relevant blood tests, and the patient can then be seen in a follow-up diabetic clinic with the appropriately trained nurse.

As with everything else you do, it is always useful to have a clear understanding of why the problems might occur and what you are looking for when you perform the task. This chapter will explain some of the underlying reasons for problems in the feet of diabetic patients and will identify how you can check for these to determine the patient's risk of ulceration.

AN OVERVIEW OF DIABETES

Diabetes mellitus is the medical term used to encompass Type 1 and Type 2 diabetes. The word diabetes is Greek in origin, and means siphon (to pass through), referring to the glucose passing into the blood and urine. Mellitus is Latin in origin, and means honeyed or sweet. In medieval times, diabetes would be diagnosed by tasting the patient's urine to see if it was sweet. Fortunately, we have moved on a little in our testing techniques!

Diabetes is a rapidly increasing problem and is associated with many complications – including heart disease, blindness and amputation – so the implications for the health services are huge, and urgent action is needed to try to halt the epidemic.

Figures for 2022–2023 show an estimated 5.6 million people with diabetes in the UK. This figure is the highest yet recorded and included 1.2 million people who were still to be diagnosed and were unaware that they had it (Diabetes UK 2024a).

People without diabetes have a pancreas that produces a hormone called insulin. We need glucose in its simplest form to provide our cells with energy so that they can work efficiently. When we ingest glucose

DOI: 10.4324/9781003460381-22

or more complex carbohydrates that are broken down into glucose, the insulin acts like a key to facilitate the entry of glucose through the cell wall and into the cell.

While we currently still refer to Type 1 and Type 2 diabetes, there may be as many as five different types, and more accurate diagnosis at an earlier stage could give doctors a better idea of how it will develop over time, allowing them to predict and treat complications before they develop (Ahlqvist et al. 2018). More research is needed to clearly differentiate between these types, so for now we'll just consider the two types we are familiar with.

TYPE 1 DIABETES

This is the less common form of diabetes, accounting for only about 10% of cases. In people with this condition, the specialised cells in the pancreas are destroyed by the body's own immune system. This is called autoimmune disease, whereby the body produces immunity to its own cells. The pancreas is then unable to produce insulin. The onset of this type of diabetes usually occurs in younger people and symptoms tend to appear suddenly. At present, the cause of Type 1 diabetes is not clear, and there is no way to prevent it. The only treatment is to take insulin by injection or via an insulin pump for life, but there is a lot of very promising research in this area, and developments such as cell transplantation and the artificial pancreas are already becoming a reality. The artificial pancreas (known as the hybrid closed loop system) will be provided in 2024 for many thousands of children and adults with Type 1 diabetes. This device continually monitors a person's blood glucose and then automatically adjusts the amount of insulin given to them through a pump (NHS England 2024).

Another development is the islet cell transplant (islet cells in the pancreas produce insulin), which can be performed on patients who meet a specific set of criteria, as a minor procedure under local anaesthetic. This has been available since 2015 in the UK. This option is more limited because of the scarcity of donor islets, so the research is now looking at ways of growing new insulin producing cells in the lab (Diabetes UK 2021a).

TYPE 2 DIABETES

In this situation, the pancreas may not produce enough insulin so that not all the glucose can get into the cells. Alternatively, the pancreas may produce enough insulin but it appears to be resisted by the effect of excess body fat. When there is not enough insulin, the body cannot cope with the glucose ('impaired glucose tolerance'). The result of this is that the specialised cells in the pancreas (beta cells) work harder to produce more insulin and eventually become worn out so they are no longer able to produce enough insulin. Factors such as obesity, sedentary lifestyle, ageing, genetics and smoking can all predispose to Type 2 diabetes. The onset usually occurs in older people, but is increasingly seen in much younger people, presumably due to the increase in obesity in that age group. Symptoms tend to appear gradually, and the patient can be treated with diet, tablets and/or insulin.

Research has shown that about 50% of cases of Type 2 diabetes can be prevented or delayed by maintaining a healthy weight, eating well and being active (Diabetes UK 2023). This is quite a mind-blowing statistic!

Obesity is the single biggest risk factor for diabetes, accounting for 80–85% of the overall risk of developing Type 2 diabetes, and it is the global rise in obesity that appears to be fuelling the current epidemic. Currently the two most promising areas for weight loss in obese or overweight patients with Type 2 diabetes are low-carbohydrate diets and very low-calorie diets (Moseley 2016; Diabetes UK 2021b). It should be noted, however, that this type of diet is not suitable for patients with Type 1 diabetes or for children. Furthermore, it is a short-term effective option and should not be seen as the diet for everyone.

An NHS Diabetes Prevention Programme in England which is based on healthy living appears to have resulted in a 7% reduction in new diagnoses of Type 2 diabetes between 2018 and 2019, saving about 18,000 people from the disease, as well as saving the NHS a considerable amount of money on treating the disease (NHS England 2022).

The main problem with diabetes is that it results in a greater amount of circulating glucose in the arteries and less in the body cells, where it is really needed. This can result in various symptoms.

ACTIVITY

List as many things as you can think of that may be *symptoms* of diabetes. You may need to look these up.

Check your list against the list given in Box 17.1.

HOW DOES DIABETES CAUSE FOOT PROBLEMS?

Diabetic foot disease is still the most common cause of hospital admission in diabetic patients (see Figure 17.1). This is because of two main factors: peripheral neuropathy and peripheral vascular disease.

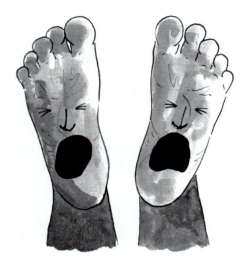

Figure 17.1 Screaming feet

Peripheral neuropathy

Research shows an overall prevalence of diabetic neuropathy of 28.5% in people with diabetes, rising to 44% in patients aged between 70–79. (Feldman 2024)

Peripheral neuropathy is nerve damage that is caused by increased glucose circulating in the blood. The glucose injures the walls of the arteries and prevents essential nutrients from reaching the nerves. Nerves carry messages of sensation and pain. If the nerves are damaged, patients may experience symptoms such as numbness, tingling, burning or stabbing pain, extreme sensitivity to touch, skin, hair or nail changes, and a lack of coordination. The patient may lose sensation in the feet and may not know if they have an injury.

This loss of protective sensation (LOPS) is the single most important risk factor in the development of a foot ulcer.

Severe neuropathy can also cause a rare deformity called Charcot foot. The bones in the foot become weak and can fracture, and if the patient continues to walk on these weakened or fractured bones, the foot will change shape and will develop the characteristic 'rocker bottom'. Sometimes there may be a deformity on the side of the foot as well (see Figure 17.2). The protrusion forms a point of increased pressure, and can ulcerate and become infected easily.

Suspect acute Charcot **arthropathy** if the foot is abnormally red, warm, swollen or deformed.

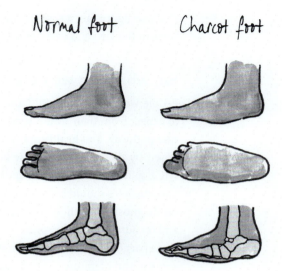

Figure 17.2 Charcot foot

If Charcot foot is suspected, it necessitates an urgent referral to confirm the diagnosis and early intervention to avoid permanent foot deformity, ulceration and possible limb loss (Vopat et al. 2018).

Peripheral vascular disease

Diabetes is strongly associated with **atherosclerosis**, which is the narrowing of the arteries due to fatty deposits (atheroma). Associated risk factors include hypertension, smoking and hyperlipidaemia. Blood flow is reduced, and skin with a poor blood supply is more prone to damage and does not heal well.

Some shocking statistics

An estimated 10% – or around 450,000 – of diabetes patients will develop a foot ulcer at some time in their lives, with more than 7,000 diabetes-related amputations occurring in the UK every year (Mackenzie 2017). A large percentage of these amputations are preventable because they begin as foot ulcers which are avoidable and can be treated if picked up early.

Approximately £650 million is spent each year on foot ulcers and amputations, and of people who do develop an ulcer, 50% will die within five years, while of those who have an amputation, up to 70% will die within five years (NHS England 2019).

These figures are a shocking indictment of the care of people with diabetes in the UK, and every effort must be made to reverse this situation.

So, what can we do about it?

People with diabetes should know how to look after their feet and what to expect from their health service. There needs to be an integrated foot-care pathway, and healthcare workers need to be more aware of the risks posed by diabetic foot disease and of the need for annual checks. The NICE guidance (NICE 2015 updated 2019) recommends that adults who have diabetes should have their risk of developing a foot problem assessed on diagnosis, and then at least annually, when any foot problems arise and on admission to hospital.

As part of its 'Putting Feet First' campaign, Diabetes UK has produced some useful literature for patients and health professionals (Diabetes UK 2018). These provide background information and an effective foot care pathway. There is a clear flow chart in which risk is identified as low, moderate, high or active, and each risk level is defined and accompanied by an action plan. Diabetes UK has coined the phrase 'Fast Track for a Foot Attack' to emphasise the seriousness of new or increasing symptoms, and to promote the concept of rapid access for treatment by a specialist multidisciplinary team to promote faster healing and fewer amputations.

All nurses and HCAs who are involved in the management of patients with diabetes should be able to perform a diabetic foot check and should receive training for this from a recognised organisation or qualified podiatrist.

CHECKING THE FEET OF THE DIABETIC PATIENT: THE PROCEDURE

You can download the Diabetic HA4 Skills for Health Framework to use as a checklist for your competencies (Skills for Health 2021).

The aims of the diabetic foot examination are to:

- detect risk factors for ulceration;
- classify the risk as low, increased or high;
- refer appropriately; and
- give feedback to the nurse or doctor.

1 Confirm the identity of the patient.
2 Obtain informed verbal consent.

3 Prior to the patient removing their footwear, have a good look at it. Does it fit well? Is it enclosed? Does it support the foot well? Is it 'breathable'?

4 Check the history – ask the following questions:

- Have you ever had a foot ulcer?
- Have you seen any cuts or blisters that you didn't feel?
- Do you have any discomfort or altered sensation in your feet or legs, either at rest or when walking?
- Do you have any problems looking after your feet?

5 The patient should be seated comfortably on an examination couch and legs should be bare from the knees down. Any socks, stockings or bandages must be removed.

6 Wash your hands.

7 Inspection:

- Inspect the shape of the foot. Is there any evidence of deformity or a Charcot foot (see Figure 17.2)?
- Inspect the skin on all areas of the lower legs and feet. Check behind the heels and over the balls of the feet for dry, cracking skin and fissures. Check between the toes and examine each toenail for length, colour, thickness, debris, odour and separation of the nail bed. Note the character and colour of the skin on the legs and the feet. Record any changes in colour and texture of the skin. Check for the presence of varicose veins or **hemosiderosis** (brown staining over the ankle area). This can indicate poor venous return and lead to oedema in the lower legs, with an increased risk of venous ulcers.
- Note any bunions or calluses and record their location, size and colour, as these could indicate areas of mechanical stress or pre-ulcer formation.
- Check the *skin temperature* by using the back of the hand on both legs, working down from the tibia (underneath the knee) to the toes. Normally, the leg is warmer at the tibia and gets cooler at the toes. Patients with neuropathy have no change in temperature or the toes may feel abnormally warm to touch, and may look red and shiny because of dilation of the capillaries in the toes.

8 Vascular assessment:

- Check the *capillary filling time* by pressing the pulp of the big toe until it blanches, and then release. It will normally take between zero and five

Essential Knowledge and Skills for Healthcare Assistants

> It is helpful to use two or three fingers to feel for the pulses. For the dorsalis pedis pulse, press lightly on top of the foot, starting just below the gap between the big toe and second toe. Work your way up the foot in line with the normal route of the artery (see Figure 17.4). For the posterior tibial pulse, flex the patient's foot and cup your three fingers around the inside ankle bone. Take your time doing this. Foot pulses can be difficult to feel!

seconds for **reperfusion** to occur, when the toe will become pink again. Delayed refill can be an indicator of arterial narrowing and ischaemia, and should be documented.

- Feel for the *dorsalis pedis pulse* on the top of the foot and the *posterior tibial pulse* behind the inside ankle bone (see Figure 17.3).

9   If you are unable to feel the pulses, use a Doppler probe (8 Mhz) and ultrasound gel to try to locate them. Apply the probe at about 45–70° and find the area that provides the clearest audible pulsatile sound (see Figure 17.5).

10 Sensory assessment:

- Use a 10g monofilament. Show the patient it is not sharp by applying it to the patient's hand first.
- Ask the patient to shut their eyes and then gently apply the monofilament to the foot in at least five places as indicated (see Figure 17.6). Try

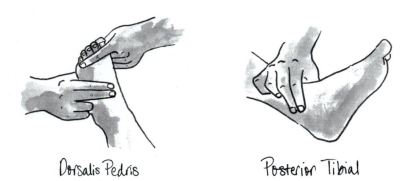

Figure 17.3 Foot pulses

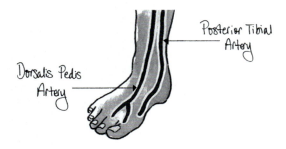

Figure 17.4 Arteries in the foot

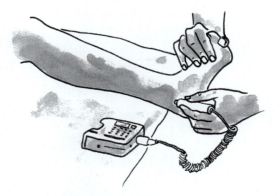

Figure 17.5 Using the Doppler to locate the posterior tibial pulse

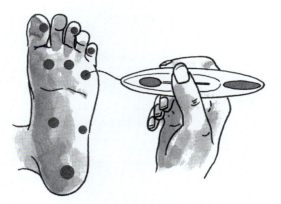

Figure 17.6 Checking for sensory perception using a monofilament

to do this randomly so that the patient is not able to predict where you will touch the foot. You should press the filament on the foot until it just bends, and then release. Ask the patient to tell you every time they feel the filament. Avoid callused areas or hard skin.
- Ideally, use disposable monofilaments, but if these are not available, make sure that the filament is cleaned with a disinfectant wipe between each patient, and do not use for more than ten patients in one session. Monofilaments should be left for at least 24 hours between sessions to recover their 'buckling strength', and should be replaced every six months.
- Record how many times the patient feels the monofilament. If they feel three out of five touches, record this as 3/5 on the template (see Table 17.1).
- If the patient is unable to feel the filament at one or more sites, the diagnosis of LOPS is made, and must be recorded appropriately on the diabetic foot clinic template.

Table 17.1 Example of diabetic foot examination template for documentation

	Right	Left	Comments
Previous foot ulcer	Yes/No	Yes/No	
Amputation	Yes/No	Yes/No	
Deformity	Yes/No	Yes/No	
Presence of callus	Yes/No	Yes/No	
Skin condition	Normal/ Abnormal	Normal/ Abnormal	
Skin colour	Normal/ Abnormal	Normal/ Abnormal	
Hair growth	Normal/ Abnormal	Normal/ Abnormal	
Nail disorders	Yes/No	Yes/No	
Footwear	Suitable/ Unsuitable	Suitable/ Unsuitable	
Dorsalis pedis pulse	Present/ Absent	Present/ Absent	
Posterior tibial pulse	Present/ Absent	Present/ Absent	
Positive monofilament test	/5	/5	
Self-care capacity		Good Moderate Poor	
Risk category		Low Moderate High Active	
Action taken			
Advice given			
Review date			

Examining the feet of people with diabetes

11 Wash hands.

12 Identify the risk of ulceration and inform the patient. Explain the follow-up or referral procedure according to the identified risk (see Table 17.2).

13 Advise the patient on home foot care. Provide Diabetes UK leaflets on foot care (available to order on the Diabetes UK website), and give contact numbers for the patient to use in case of any changes or concerns.

14 Document all results in the diabetic clinic foot examination template. EMIS and Vision platforms will have specific templates for this, but if you need to develop one of your own, you may find the example in Table 17.1 useful as a guide).

Table 17.2 Classifying the risk of ulceration (NICE 2023)

Risk	Action
Low risk *No risk factors present* except callus alone (e.g. no loss of sensation, no signs of peripheral vascular disease and no other risk factors).	Annual foot assessments. Emphasise the risk of developing problems and the importance of foot care. Provide appropriate leaflets and emergency contact numbers, and encourage the patient to return if they experience any changes or problems with their feet.
Moderate risk *One risk factor present* (e.g. loss of sensation or signs of peripheral vascular disease without callus or deformity).	Refer to podiatrist – patient should be seen within 6–8 weeks. Emphasise the risk of developing problems and the importance of foot care. Provide appropriate leaflets and emergency contact numbers, and encourage the patient to return if they experience any changes or problems with their feet. Review in 3–6 months.

(Continued)

Table 17.2 (*Continued*) Classifying the risk of ulceration (NICE 2023)

Risk	Action
High risk *Previous ulceration or amputation, or on renal replacement therapy, or more than one risk factor present* (e.g. loss of sensation or signs of peripheral vascular disease with callus or deformity).	Seek advice from diabetic nurse or GP. Refer to podiatrist – to be seen in 1–3 months, depending on need. Emphasise the risk of developing problems and the importance of foot care. Provide appropriate leaflets and emergency contact numbers, and encourage the patient to return if they experience any changes or problems with their feet. Review with GP or diabetic nurse every 1–2 months if there is no immediate concern, or every 1–2 weeks if there is immediate concern.
Active *Presence of active ulceration, spreading infection* (e.g. critical ischaemia, gangrene or unexplained hot, red, swollen foot with or without pain, painful peripheral neuropathy, acute Charcot foot).	Seek immediate advice from diabetic nurse or GP. Patient should be referred within one working day to the multidisciplinary foot care service according to local protocols and pathways. Provide appropriate leaflets and emergency contact numbers.

There are other tools available that can be used to detect loss of sensation:

- *VibraTip* is a small battery-operated vibrating tool that may provide an alternative to the monofilament in the future, but NICE medical technology guidance (NICE 2014 updated 2015) advises that further research is needed before it can be used more widely in the NHS. This advice remains unchanged at time of writing the third edition of this book (2024). Some recent research does now suggest that an abnormal VibraTip result is almost always associated with LOPS, but also advises use of the VibraTip in conjunction with the monofilament to improve sensitivity (Pasangha et al. 2021).

- *Tuning fork (128Hz)*: NICE (2023) only advises the use of monofilaments, so tuning forks are not included in the procedure previously described, but there are many useful videos available on YouTube that show how to use the tuning fork to test for neuropathy if you need to know this.

> Any doubt? Not sure about your findings? Unable to feel or hear the pulses?
>
> If you have *any* concerns about your patient, however small, *always* discuss them with the registered nurse or doctor.

ENCOURAGING PATIENTS TO LOOK AFTER THEIR FEET

We know that people with diabetes who take good care of their feet and protect their feet from injury are much less likely to develop foot ulcers. Work in partnership with your patient to provide them with the appropriate information. Involve them (and their partner or carer) in any decision-making, provide contact numbers for them to ring in case of any problems, and always back up any verbal information with written information.

AFTERCARE ADVICE FOR YOUR PATIENT

You can type out the following advice and make it into a leaflet for your patient or use a leaflet from Diabetes UK (Diabetes UK 2024b).

- Look for and report any changes.
- Never try to deal with corns, calluses or verrucae yourself.
- Use moisturiser regularly (but not between the toes).
- Always cut nails straight across and never down at the sides.
- Wash feet daily and dry carefully.
- Never walk barefoot.
- Always wear socks with shoes (and sandals!).

- Shoes should fit well and be wide enough to reduce the risk of rubbing.
- Always feel inside shoes before putting them on.
- Check bath temperature before stepping in.
- Avoid the use of hot water bottles or electric blankets.
- Never sit too close to a fire.

Box 17.1 Common symptoms of diabetes

> - Urinary frequency – usually worse at night.
> - Increased thirst.
> - Increased hunger.
> - Weight loss.
> - Tiredness.
> - Recurrent infections.
> - Candidiasis (thrush) infection.
> - Blurred vision.
> - Erectile dysfunction.
> - Wounds that won't heal.
> - Numbness, tingling or pain in the feet or hands.

Now try the following quiz. You can check back in the text for the answers.

DIABETES QUIZ

1. Where is insulin produced in the body?
2. What are the differences between Type 1 diabetes and Type 2 diabetes?
3. What is the single biggest risk factor for Type 2 diabetes?
4. What is peripheral neuropathy?
5. What is peripheral vascular disease?
6. Where is the dorsalis pedis pulse located?
7. Where is the posterior tibial pulse located?
8. How many points should you test on each foot with the monofilament?
9. When is LOPS diagnosed?
10. What will you do if the patient is at 'moderate risk' of ulceration?

TIME TO REFLECT

Using a framework for reflection (see Chapter 2), try reflecting on a consultation when you watched or performed a diabetic foot examination.

How did it go? What did you learn?

How does a frog feel when he has a bad toe? Unhoppy!

REFERENCES

Ahlqvist, E., Storm, P., Käräjämäki, A. et al. (2018) Novel subgroups of adult-onset diabetes and their association with outcomes: A data-driven cluster analysis of six variables. *Diabetes and Endocrinology* 6(5): 361–369. https://www.ncbi.nlm.nih.gov/pubmed/29503172 (accessed September 18, 2024).

Diabetes UK (2018) *Putting Feet First*. https://www.diabetes.org.uk/support-us/campaign/other-campaigns/putting-feet-first (accessed September 29, 2024).

Diabetes UK (2021a) *Islet Transplants: Our Research Changes National Guidelines*. https://www.diabetes.org.uk/about-us/news-and-views/islet-transplant-guidance-changed (accessed September 26, 2024).

Diabetes UK (2021b) *Low Carb Diets Position Statement for Professionals 2021*. https://www.diabetes.org.uk/for-professionals/supporting-your-patients/clinical-recommendations-for-professionals/low-carb-diets-for-people-with-diabetes (accessed September 26, 2024).

Diabetes UK (2023) *How to Prevent Type 2 Diabetes*. https://www.diabetes.org.uk/diabetes-the-basics/types-of-diabetes/type-2/preventing (accessed September 18, 2024).

Diabetes UK (2024a) *How Many People in the UK Have Diabetes?* https://www.diabetes.org.uk/about-us/about-the-charity/our-strategy/statistics (accessed September 18, 2024).

Diabetes UK (2024b) *How to Look After Your Feet*. https://www.diabetes.org.uk/guide-to-diabetes/complications/feet/taking-care-of-your-feet (accessed September 29, 2024).

Feldman, E. (2024) *Epidemiology and Classification of Diabetic Neuropathy*. https://www.uptodate.com/contents/epidemiology-and-classification-of-diabetic-neuropathy (accessed September 27, 2024).

Mackenzie, P. (2017) *Diabetes Footcare Project 1: Pathway Development*. https://www.england.nhs.uk/north/wp-content/uploads/

sites/5/2018/05/NWCSN_Diabetes_Footcare_Final_Report_2017–1. pdf (accessed September 27, 2024).

Moseley, M. (2016) *The Blood Sugar Diet*. https://thebloodsugardiet.com (accessed September 26, 2024).

NHS England (2019) *Local NHS Team Sets the National Standard for Improving Footcare for Patients with Diabetes*. https://www.england. nhs.uk/south-east/2019/04/02/local-nhs-team-sets-the-national-standard-for-improving-foot-care-for-patients-with-diabetes (accessed September 27, 2024).

NHS England (2022) *NHS Prevention Programme Cuts Chances of Type 2 Diabetes for Thousands*. https://www.england.nhs.uk/2022/03/ nhs-prevention-programme-cuts-chances-of-type-2-diabetes-for-thousands (accessed September 26, 2024).

NHS England (2024) *NHS Rolls Out Artificial Pancreas in World First Move*. https://www.england.nhs.uk/2024/04/nhs-rolls-out-artificial-pancreas-in-world-first-move (accessed September 26, 2024).

NICE (2014 updated 2015) *VibraTip for Testing Vibration Perception to Detect Diabetic Peripheral Neuropathy. Medical Technologies Guidance*. https://www.nice.org.uk/guidance/mtg22 (accessed September 29, 2024).

NICE (2015 updated 2019) *NICE Guideline NG19 Diabetic Foot Problems: Prevention and Management*. https://www.nice.org.uk/ guidance/ng19 (accessed November 25, 2024).

NICE (2023) *Diabetic Foot Problems: Prevention and Management*. https://www.nice.org.uk/guidance/ng19/evidence/b-risk-assessment-models-and-tools-for-predicting-the-development-of-diabetic-foot-problems-and-foot-review-frequency-pdf-6953995119 (accessed November 4, 2024).

Pasangha, E., George, B., Jayalakshmi, V. et al. (2021) The utility of Vibratip in accurate identification in loss of protective sensation in the contralateral foot of patients admitted with a diabetic foot ulcer. *Diabetes & Metabolic Syndrome: Clinical Research & Reviews*. https:// www.sciencedirect.com/science/article/abs/pii/S1871402121000977 (accessed September 29, 2024).

Skills for Health (2021) *Diab HA4 Assess the Feet of Individuals with Diabetes and Provide Advice on Maintaining Healthy Feet and Managing Foot Problems*. https://tools.skillsforhealth.org.uk/ competence-details/html/4337 (accessed September 29, 2024).

Vopat, M., Nentwig, M., Chong, A.C.M. et al. (2018) Initial diagnosis and management for acute Charcot neuroarthropathy. *Kansas Journal of Medicine* 11(14): 114–119. https://www.ncbi.nlm.nih.gov/ pmc/articles/PMC6276967 (accessed September 27, 2024).

The skin and the healing process

Basic wound care

18

As with all other clinical procedures, before you can embark on basic wound care, you must attend a recognised training course, have written evidence of your competence and have a clear protocol in place with care plans that have been drawn up by the registered nurse for each patient. A care plan does not need to be a long, complicated document, but can be a simple set of instructions on the computer notes, identifying things such as the duration of treatment, the type of dressing to be used and when to refer to the nurse for advice.

You should have knowledge of the skin and how it heals, and you must understand the principles of the Aseptic Non-Touch Technique (ANTT), which is discussed later in this chapter.

SKIN ANATOMY

Skin is the largest organ of the body – about two square metres in volume, weighing about six pounds. It basically keeps the outside out and the inside in! There are three layers in skin, and each layer has a specific function.

Epidermis

This is the outermost layer that protects the body from the elements. It prevents the entry of harmful microorganisms and can dispose of harmful pathogens. It prevents loss of fluid and contains melanin cells. These cells give the skin its colour and protect the body from ultraviolet light.

Dermis

This is the layer of skin under the epidermis containing the nerve endings, blood vessels, oil glands and sweat glands. It also contains collagen and elastin, which give skin its strength and elasticity, sadly lacking as we

DOI: 10.4324/9781003460381-23

get older! The dermis regulates the body temperature through sweating and vasodilation (widening) and constriction (narrowing) of the capillaries near the surface. Pre-vitamin D_3 is formed in the dermis during exposure to sunlight, and this is then rearranged to form vitamin D_3. This is necessary to regulate the concentration of calcium and phosphate in the bloodstream, promoting healthy bones.

Subcutaneous fat

This is the loose **connective tissue** largely made up of fat cells called adipocytes. It stores energy as lipids, helps keep the body warm, acts as a shock absorber, holds the skin to the underlying tissues and houses the hair follicles.

THE PHYSIOLOGY OF WOUND HEALING

It is worth stopping to think sometimes about everything that is going on in your body without you even realising. When you cut a finger or if you sustain a much larger wound, the body sets to work immediately to clean and heal the wound. It is quite amazing how efficient the body can be at looking after us, even when we may not be very good at it ourselves!

Haemostasis (meaning the stopping of blood flow) is the body's natural response to injury. The damaged blood vessels temporarily constrict to stop the bleeding. Activation of the clotting mechanism then occurs, resulting in the release of chemicals called clotting factors, which are identified by the Roman numerals I–XIII. Factor I, called fibrinogen, is converted to solid strands of protein called fibrin. The platelets become sticky and clump around the injured tissue. These are then reinforced by the strands of fibrin, forming platelet plugs, sealing the injury and initiating healing.

Stage 1: the inflammatory phase

This lasts between zero and five days, and begins the healing response. There may be heat, redness, swelling and pain at this stage. White blood cells collect in large numbers at the site of injury, and proceed to remove dead tissue, foreign material and pathogens from the wound.

At this stage, yellow **slough** may appear on the wound surface and there may be redness around the wound. This is normal *at this stage*, and should not be confused with infection.

Stage 2: proliferation/granulation phase

This usually goes on from days 3–14, and may overlap with the first phase. This is an important phase in wounds where there is skin loss. Tiny new blood vessels (capillaries) form in the dermis to supply blood with essential nutrients and oxygen, and the wound bed granulation can then begin. The healing 'granulating' tissue should appear to be bright red, 'beefy' and moist. If the wound bed is moist, new pale pink skin cells (epithelial cells) can multiply and migrate across the wound bed in a process called **epithelialisation**. This process is delicate and easily hindered if the wound bed is not moist or if it is exposed to any further trauma during wound cleansing or during the removal of old dressings.

Stage 3: maturation phase

This usually begins at about day 7 and can last up to 12 months. There is a progressive reduction in the blood supply to the scar. Collagen fibres become bigger and reoriented to improve the strength of the new skin. The scar becomes paler and should eventually flatten and soften.

TYPES OF HEALING

Primary healing

This is also called *first intention healing*, and this occurs when the wound closes by the coming together of the wound edges, either spontaneously or with intervention such as with sutures or clips.

Secondary healing

This occurs where there has been tissue loss. The wound heals by the process of epithelialisation (see under stage 2 as previously described) and wound contraction. There is no surgical intervention.

ACTIVITY

There are many different factors that can affect the healing process.

List as many things as you can you think of that may delay healing.

How could this affect patient care?

Check your answers in Box 18.1.

PROBLEMS IN THE HEALING PROCESS

An essential part of basic wound care is the ability to recognise what is normal and when there may be problems.

Clinical signs of infection

All wounds will have microorganisms present, but this does not necessarily mean that the wound is infected. Routine wound swabbing may therefore provide erroneous and misleading results.

Wound infection occurs when there are sufficient pathogens present in the wound so that they cause damage to the body tissue, and ultimately provoke a host reaction. Pathogens can be bacteria, viruses or fungal organisms, but they are usually bacteria in infected skin wounds.

Wound swabbing should only be carried out when there are clinical signs of infection.

There are some important signs to look out for that may indicate problems in the healing process or possible infection, and these should always be reported to the registered nurse or doctor immediately.

Signs indicating possible infection include the following.

- Wound increasing or not reducing in size.
- Increasing pain.
- Heat.
- Erythema (redness).
- Cellulitis.
- Oedema (swelling).
- Wound breakdown.
- Malodour (bad smell).
- Increased **exudate** (fluid leaking from the wound).
- Fragile granulation tissue – wound bleeds easily.
- **Systemic** signs of fever and **malaise**, pyrexia.

TAKING A WOUND SWAB: THE PROCEDURE

Swabbing appears to be a straightforward task, but if done badly can lead to an incorrect diagnosis and inappropriate treatment, delayed healing and all the subsequent effects that may have on the patient.

The decision on whether to perform a swab should be made by the registered nurse or doctor, but the task may be performed by the HCA.

Always collect the swab before any topical or systemic antibiotics are started. If the patient has had an **antimicrobial** dressing in place (see Table 18.1), delay taking the swab because the microbial count will be reduced and you will have a meaningless result.

Follow these simple steps to ensure accurate sampling.

1   Explain the procedure to the patient and obtain informed consent.
2   Decontaminate your hands and put on gloves.
3   Irrigate the wound to remove slough, **necrotic** tissue or dried exudate using tap water or sterile saline. Irrigating may also reduce the risk of introducing erroneous organisms into the specimen. The wound must be moistened if it appears dry, as this will improve the 'catch' of the swab. There is little to be gained from swabbing a dry wound. Alternatively, the swab tip can be moistened with sterile saline prior to performing the swab. Use a sterile cotton or rayon-tipped swab in a charcoal medium.
4   Move the swab across the wound bed in a zigzag motion at the same time as rotating the swab between the fingers, covering as large an area of the wound as possible, working away from the area that is cleanest. Include material from the wound bed and wound margin but avoid touching the swab on the surrounding skin. (Titman Revised 2023).
5   Immediately place the swab back into the container with the transport medium.
6   Remove your gloves and decontaminate your hands.
7   Label the sample correctly and complete the necessary documentation to send with it. Include any relevant comments about the patient's general condition, type of wound, etc.
8   Record in the patient notes.
9   Ensure transport of the swab to the laboratory as soon as possible (ideally within four hours).

Choosing the wound dressing

Each patient should have a clear care plan drawn up by the registered nurse at the initial assessment of the patient and their wound. The care plan will specify the type of dressing to be used and the frequency of dressing change. Most patients should be reviewed by the registered nurse regularly throughout the course of their treatment, but the frequency will depend on the severity of the wound. Always refer to the nurse if there are any problems or changes in the patient's condition.

Table 18.1 Types of dressings*

Category	Qualities	Suitable for	Points to consider	Example
Simple contact	Non-absorbent, **low adherence**. Sometimes requires a secondary dressing.	Low exuding wounds. Fragile, delicate skin. Skin tears in the elderly.	Not suitable for heavily exuding wounds.	Atrauman Urgotul Mepitel Interpose Mepore
Semipermeable film membranes	Permeable to water vapour and oxygen but **impermeable** to liquid. Transparent.	Wounds with little or no exudate (e.g. minor operation wounds healing by primary intention).	Not suitable for heavily exuding wounds.	C-view Tegaderm film Opsite
Hydrocolloids	Absorbs water to form a gel – maintains a moist environment. Can facilitate rehydration and **debridement** of dry sloughy or necrotic wounds.	Granulating or necrotic wounds. Low to moderate exudate.	Avoid in diabetic foot wounds. Caution in infected wounds, as hydrocolloids can encourage the growth of anaerobic bacteria.	Hydrocoll Comfeel-Plus Duoderm Granuflex
Alginates	Will change to a gel in the presence of exudate. Highly absorbent. Haemostatic (stops bleeding). Debriding action. Requires secondary dressing.	Lightly exuding or bleeding wounds. Acute surgical wounds. Cavity wounds.	Not suitable for dry or necrotic wounds. Should not be used with creams or ointments, as these may prevent the gelling process. Should never be left in a wound – all traces should be removed. Can cause **maceration** and **excoriation** of surrounding skin.	Kaltostat Sorbsan

Table 18.1 *(Continued)* Types of dressings*

Category	Qualities	Suitable for	Points to consider	Example
Hydrofibre	Absorbs and interacts with wound exudate to form a soft **hydrophilic** gas permeable gel. Traps bacteria. Requires a secondary dressing.	Exuding lesions.	Very lightly exuding wounds may need to be moistened with sterile water or saline before application of the dressing. Not suitable for dry necrotic wounds.	Aquacel-Extra
Silver dressings	Antimicrobial action.	For critically colonised and infected wounds.	If no improvement is noted within two weeks, replace with non-silver product.	Acticoat 3 or 7
Foams	Good absorption. Provide mechanical protection. May be used as a secondary dressing.	Exuding wounds (vary in absorption according to product used). May be beneficial in **hypergranulating** tissue.	Not for dry wounds. Always select appropriate size.	Activheal Tegaderm foam Biatain
Odour-absorbent dressings	Absorb odour.	Malignant **fungating** wounds where there is an anaerobic infection with unpleasant odour.	Avoid unnecessary use.	Clinisorb Carboflex
Paraffin gauze	Reduces adherence of the dressing to the granulating wound. Requires secondary dressing.	Burns, ulcers, traumatic injuries, skin grafts.	Beware of maceration to surrounding skin in a heavily exuding wound. May become adherent if left on for too long.	Jelonet

(Continued)

Table 18.1 (*Continued*) Types of dressings*

Category	Qualities	Suitable for	Points to consider	Example
Cadoxemer iodine	Absorbs exudate. Debriding action. Antimicrobial action. Requires secondary dressing.	Lightly exuding wounds at risk of infection.	Avoid in pregnant patients or thyroid disorders, or on lithium therapy. Take care in patients with iodine sensitivity. May cause stinging or burning. Treatment should not exceed three months.	Inadine Iodoflex
Honey	Antibacterial action. Debriding and anti-inflammatory properties. Maintains moist wound bed. Reduces odour. Stimulates growth of new capillaries and skin cells. May require secondary dressing.	Open wounds healing by secondary intention.	May increase exudate. May cause stinging or burning.	Algivon Mesitran Medihoney
Zinc paste bandages	Cooling and soothing. Provide a moist wound environment.	**Varicose eczema.**	Must be applied correctly (i.e., pleated or layered), as it will tighten when it dries.	Steripaste Zipzoc Viscopaste

* Follow the manufacturer's guidelines to apply the dressing correctly.

The skin and the healing process

Before deciding on the wound dressing, the nurse should consider:

- the patient, their health status, environment and mobility;
- the wound type, size and cause;
- allergies or intolerances;
- dressing efficacy (based on evidence);
- cost;
- acceptability to patient and prescriber; and
- local wound care formulary.

> Remember, dressings should be prescribed for individual patients and are single-use only. They should not be resealed and used again.

ACTIVITY

Considering what you now know about the skin and the healing process, can you list the qualities of the ideal wound dressing? Check your answers in Box 18.2.

There are many different wound dressings, and intelligent use of the appropriate dressing can speed up the healing process. The choice of dressing should always be guided by the local wound care formulary, as this will be based on current, available, unbiased and robust evidence.

ACTIVITY

Look up your local wound care formulary or contact your local tissue viability nurse, who will tell you where you can obtain a copy from. You must be able to justify the use of dressings that are not included in the local formulary. Table 18.1 gives a list of dressings as listed in some wound care formularies, and outlines their qualities and suitability for various wounds.

How do you reduce the risk of infection when performing a simple wound dressing?

Most healthcare-acquired infections are entirely preventable (as we saw in Chapter 10).

The main infection risk to the patient is the health worker – that's you! The level of risk can be minimised by using an effective aseptic technique during any invasive procedure, such as when performing a wound dressing. ANTT is a framework for aseptic practice that was designed in 2013 and which has been developed and disseminated by the Association for Safe Aseptic Practice (Association for Safe Aseptic Practice ASAP 2024) to improve the standard of aseptic technique in clinical practice. ANTT is now the national standard aseptic technique in England, Wales and Australia, and is used in more than 30 countries.

Asepsis is usually defined as the 'absence of microorganisms', but this is not truly achievable in typical healthcare settings. On this basis, the ANTT principle defines asepsis as 'free from pathogenic organisms in sufficient numbers to cause infection'.

Asepsis is achieved by 'key part' and 'key site' protection; key parts refer to things such as the tip of a syringe or the wound side of a dressing, and key sites refer to things such as open wounds and surgical incisions or any portal of entry on a patient.

ANTT is described as 'standard ANTT' (suitable for uncomplicated, short procedures with small key parts and small key sites) and 'surgical ANTT' (suitable for procedures that are technically complex, lasting more than 20 minutes and involving large open key sites and many key parts). Standard ANTT is suitable for the type of dressings most HCAs will be performing. The aseptic field is an important component of this to ensure a controlled safe working space and help maintain asepsis. The other important components of ANTT are the non-touch technique and the use of appropriate infective precautions, such as effective hand decontamination and appropriate use of PPE. Use non-sterilised gloves if you can perform the procedure without touching key parts or key sites directly, and use sterilised gloves if you are likely to touch key parts or sites.

WOUND DRESSING: THE PROCEDURE

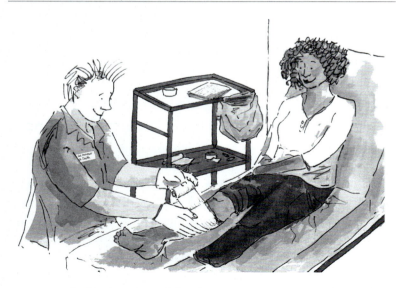

Figure 18.1 Performing a wound dressing

The skin and the healing process

You can download the National Occupational Standard CHS12 _Undertake Treatments and Dressing Related to the Care of Lesions and Wounds_ to use as a checklist for your competencies (Skills for Health 2021a).

Remember the following.

- Always use a clean trolley.
- Wash your hands before, after and at any point during the procedure if they become contaminated. Put on a disposable plastic apron.
- Use sterile equipment, fluids and dressing materials. Discard any with broken packaging or any that have passed their expiry date.
- Do not do wound dressings if you have any hand infections, boils, a sore throat or a runny nose.
- Never attempt complex dressings when you have not had appropriate training and been assessed as competent. If you are in any doubt, refer to the nurse.

1 Confirm the patient's identity and obtain informed consent before proceeding.
2 Check the care plan and patient notes from the previous appointment.
3 Prepare the patient so that they are comfortable and the area to be dressed is adequately exposed. If this involves taking off clothing, make sure the treatment area is private and the patient is provided with a dignity cover when necessary. Offer a chaperone.
4 Put on gloves to remove the dressing. Alternatively, you may ask the patient to remove the dressing themselves and offer the facility to decontaminate their hands afterwards. Another way to remove a dressing is by inserting your hand inside the bag (provided in some dressing packs) to remove the dressing, and then inverting the bag so that the dressing is contained inside. This can then be attached to the side of the trolley nearest to the patient and used as the bag to collect the dirty swabs, gloves, etc.
5 Remove gloves. Decontaminate your hands.
6 Note the condition of the wound. Seek advice from the registered nurse if the wound shows signs of any problems or if the patient reports any concerns.
7 Prepare the clean trolley. Select the appropriate dressing pack if required. Peel open and gently drop the inside pack on to the upper surface of the trolley. Open the inside pack by touching the corners only so that your hands never come into direct contact with the inside of the pack.

8 Once the sterile field is opened out on to the upper level of the trolley, other sterile items such as the dressing can be opened and gently dropped on to the field. Non-sterile items, such as irrigation pods, adhesive tape, etc., can be placed on the lower level of the trolley so that they are within reach when needed. If using saline in plastic pouches, you will need a sterile **gallipot** for the fluid, a syringe to irrigate the wound and an alcohol swab to clean the pouch.

9 Decontaminate your hands. Put on gloves.

10 Clean the wound *if necessary* by gently irrigating with warm tap water (Holman 2023) or sterile saline. Do not routinely clean wounds – they should only be cleaned if they are contaminated with foreign particles, slough or necrotic tissue. Never use gauze or cotton wool on wounds, as these may leave fibres in the wound and delay the healing process. Only ever use these to clean *around* the wound.

11 Apply the dressing(s) according to the manufacturer's instructions, without touching the side that will be in contact with the wound.

12 Apply adhesive tape if necessary (check for allergies).

13 Dispose of dressing packs and contaminated equipment in the clinical waste bin in line with your local policy.

14 Remove gloves and decontaminate your hands.

15 Make sure the patient has a new appointment if they are to be seen again, and always advise them to return sooner if they are having any problems.

16 Document your actions and observations in the patient notes.

REMOVING WOUND CLOSURES: THE PROCEDURE

You can download the National Occupational Standard CHS14 *Remove Wound Closure Materials from Individuals* to use as a checklist for your competencies (Skills for Health 2021b).

You can purchase suture removal packs, which include a sterile field, suture cutter, forceps, gauze and bag for used dressings, swabs, etc., but these may be more expensive than using individual items. Check your local wound care formulary.

Sharps should be disposed of in the sharps bin in accordance with local policy.

The skin and the healing process

Follow the preceding Steps 1–9, then proceed as follows.

10 The nurse should assess the wound prior to suture removal.
11 Remove alternate sutures to begin with in case the wound has not healed well, so that if it starts to open, there are still some sutures left **in situ**.
12 Remove the suture by pulling the knot up with forceps, and then cutting *underneath the knot closest to the skin* and pulling the suture through.
13 If there are any problems during the procedure or the patient has any discomfort, always check with the registered nurse before proceeding.
14 Dispose of the sutures in the clinical waste bag and the stitch cutter in the sharps bin.
15 Apply a dry dressing if required.
16 Remove gloves and decontaminate your hands.
17 Advise the patient to come back if they have any problems.
18 Document your actions and observations on the patient notes.

Box 18.1 Factors that may delay healing

- Infection.
- Presence of foreign object.
- Inappropriate dressing/wrong size.
- Poor dressing technique.
- Poor nutrition.
- Smoking.
- Chronic disease such as diabetes, COPD, anaemia, depression, heart disease.
- Poor circulation.
- Poor mobility.
- Social factors and environment.
- Radiotherapy/chemotherapy.
- Immunosuppression.
- Pressure.
- Medication.
- Age.

Box 18.2 Characteristics of the ideal wound dressing

- Comfortable and acceptable for the patient.
- Keep pain to a minimum.
- Maintain a moist environment where there is an open wound bed, when the wound is healing by secondary intention.
- Remove excess exudate.
- Allow the exchange of gases such as oxygen in from the air to promote healing and carbon dioxide out (waste product).
- Maintain the correct temperature to facilitate healing (not too hot or cold).
- Provide protection from further trauma.
- Prevent the entry of microorganisms.
- Leave no particles in the wound when it is removed.
- Be easily removed without causing trauma/hindering the epithelialisation of the wound.
- Be non-allergenic and non-toxic.

Now try the following quiz. You can check back in the text for the answers.

WOUND CARE QUIZ

1. What is the function of the epidermis?
2. What does haemostasis mean?
3. What do the platelets do?
4. How long does the inflammatory phase in wound healing last?
5. What happens during the proliferation/granulation phase?
6. If a wound heals by primary intention, what does this mean?
7. List five signs of infection.
8. Which parts of the wound should be sampled when performing a wound swab?
9. What type of wound would a hydrocolloid be suitable for?
10. What would you do if the patient was complaining of increased pain or exudate?

TIME TO REFLECT

Using a framework for reflection (see Chapter 2), try reflecting on a consultation when you performed a wound dressing.
How did it go, and what did you learn?

REFERENCES

Association for Safe Aseptic Practice ASAP (2024). *Aseptic Non-Touch Technique ANTT® Clinical Practice Framework.* https://www.antt.org/antt-practice-framework.html (accessed September 11, 2024).

Holman, M. (2023) *Using Tap Water Compared with Normal Saline for Cleansing Wounds in Adults: A Literature Review of the Evidence.* https://www.magonlinelibrary.com/doi/abs/10.12968/jowc.2023.32.8.507 (accessed October 6, 2024).

Skills for Health (2021a) *CHS12 Undertake Treatments and Dressings Related to the Care of Lesions and Wounds.* https://tools.skillsforhealth.org.uk/competence-details/html/4361 (accessed October 6, 2024).

Skills for Health (2021b) *CHS14 Remove Wound Closure Materials from Individuals.* https://tools.skillsforhealth.org.uk/competence-details/html/4369 (accessed October 6, 2024).

Titman, A. (Revised 2023) *Wound Swab and Culture.* https://www.exeterlaboratory.com/microbiology/wound-swab-culture (accessed October 6, 2024).

Understanding lung function and disease

Performing accurate lung function testing

Many HCAs are now being asked to perform lung function testing to assist the nurse in the chronic disease clinic, managing patients with respiratory disease. This chapter will give an overview of the anatomy and physiology of the respiratory system and common respiratory diseases to enhance your understanding and enable you to perform lung function testing more efficiently and accurately. You will need to complete a recognised course in spirometry before performing this task. Following concerns that the spirometry technique employed in many places was substandard, NHS England implemented a scheme whereby any health professional (GP, nurse or HCA) who is involved in lung function testing must be trained to a specific standard (NHS England 2020).

The Association for Respiratory Technology and Physiology (ARTP) is the only organisation to offer national, professionally recognised qualifications in respiratory function testing and spirometry in the UK, and now maintains the national register, which has been created to identify all appropriately trained and/or certified practitioners. HCAs will need to complete the foundation certificate, and this will enable them to perform the procedure competently, but not to interpret results.

WHY DO WE NEED TO BREATHE?

Breathing is something most of us take for granted and rarely think about unless we become short of breath for some reason.

Effective respiration provides us with essential oxygen, which must then be transferred from our airways into the bloodstream for distribution to all the organs and cells of the body. Oxygen is essential to help convert food into energy in our cells. This is called metabolism. Effective respiration also helps us to get rid of carbon dioxide, which is a waste product of metabolism and can become very toxic to the body if it accumulates.

When you inhale (breathe in), the **diaphragm** and muscles between the ribs (intercostal muscles) contract and make the chest cavity expand. As the chest expands, the pressure in the chest will drop, and because the outside air

DOI: 10.4324/9781003460381-24

pressure is now greater, air flows into the lungs. As you exhale (breathe out), the diaphragm and intercostal muscles relax, reducing the size of the chest cavity. This increases the pressure inside the chest so that air from inside the lungs flows to the outside. The cycle is repeated every time you breathe.

Oxygen-enriched air that we breathe in travels down the **trachea** and is then sent via the left and right **bronchus** to the bronchioles in the lungs. The bronchioles become smaller and constantly branch so that if you looked at the inside of a healthy lung, it would look something like the branches of a very dense tree in miniature. At the end of every tiny branch, there is a tiny air sac called an **alveolus** (see Figure 14.3). This is designed to maximise surface area for the exchange of gases (oxygen and carbon dioxide). From the outside, it looks like a tiny bunch of grapes wrapped in capillaries, which are tiny blood vessels. These contain deoxygenated blood – in other words, blood that has been all around the body and has used up its oxygen supply. It is sent back from the heart to the lungs, via the pulmonary artery, to collect more oxygen. The artery becomes smaller and smaller until it forms the mesh of tiny capillaries with very thin walls that are only one cell thick. The mesh of capillaries wraps intimately around the alveolus. Oxygen from the air in the alveoli can then diffuse across the cell walls and into the blood to be taken back to the left side of the heart and sent off around the body again. Carbon dioxide is transferred by the same mechanism in the opposite direction, back into the lungs and then exhaled.

Useful definitions

- *Tidal breathing*: Normal breathing, where the volume of air entering and leaving the body of a healthy adult will be about 500 ml.
- *Dead space*: The inhaled air in the airways, where no gaseous exchange can take place (usually about 150 ml).
- *Total lung capacity*: The volume of air in the lungs following maximum inspiration (usually about 6 litres).
- *Residual volume*: The air remaining in the lungs after full expiration.

LUNG DISEASE

Asthma

Asthma is a very common disease. It accounts for 2–3% of primary care consultations and is responsible for 60,000 hospital admissions per year in the UK (NICE 2023 Revised 2024).

Understanding lung function and disease

Three people will die every day in the UK from an asthma attack and someone will have a potentially life-threatening asthma attack every 10 seconds. Many of these attacks and deaths could be avoided by improving care with early and accurate diagnosis and correct treatment and education enabling self-management (Allen 2023).

So, what is it?

There is no standardised definition of the type, severity or frequency of symptoms, nor of the findings on investigation, for asthma. There are various possible symptoms, including wheeziness, breathlessness, chest tightness, cough and variable airflow obstruction. There may also be airway **hyper-responsiveness** and airway inflammation as components of the disease. It can affect people of any age, can change throughout a person's life and is characterised by attacks (or **exacerbations**), with the severity and frequency of attacks varying from person to person (NICE 2017 updated 2021).

ACTIVITY

Please *don't* try this if you already have asthma – you already know what it feels like!

For those who have never had problems breathing, try taking in a little breath. Don't breathe out, but take in another little breath, and keep doing this until you can't breathe in any more. This is what it feels like not to be able to get any more air into your lungs.

It's quite frightening, isn't it?

Asthma is very common, often misunderstood and often poorly managed. It can be very variable, very distressing and disabling, and can be life-threatening, but most of the time it can be treated.

The airways may become twitchy and constrict easily. There might be swelling or inflammation or mucus in the airways as well, which will make the airflow difficult. When the airways get smaller, the person with asthma might cough or wheeze or have difficulty breathing. Sometimes they may feel as if their chest is tight or as if there is a band around the chest. This usually happens in response to a trigger, and there are many possible triggers.

> **ACTIVITY**
>
> How many asthma triggers can you think of?
> Check your answers against those given in Box 19.1.

Asthma can occur at any age, and tends to occur most often in people with other allergies or those who have a family history of asthma. The evidence suggests that if inherited, it passes from mother to daughter and father to son (Arshad et al. 2012).

DIAGNOSIS AND TREATMENT

Various tests can be used to diagnose asthma, but there is no gold standard test available yet (NICE 2017 updated 2021).

Tests available include serial peak flow measurements, spirometry and assessment of reversibility with bronchodilators such as salbutamol. The problem with all these tests is that they are unreliable in terms of diagnosis. Testing for airway inflammation is increasingly being used for diagnosis in clinical practice, and this has been endorsed in the NICE guidance (NICE 2017 updated 2021), but will take some time to implement everywhere. It involves measuring the amount of fractional exhaled nitric oxide (FeNO), because this will be raised in patients who have inflamed airways and who are more likely to respond well to steroid treatment. A FeNO level higher than 40 makes asthma and the response to an inhaled steroid very likely, while a level lower than 20 makes it unlikely (Thomas 2018).

Asthma can be treated with various inhalers and tablets, and the treatment follows a stepwise approach (NICE 2017 updated 2021), stepping up from occasional use of a bronchodilator inhaler (this will widen the airways) to regular use of inhaled steroids that help to stop the swelling and inflammation in the airways. Some patients will need very strong doses of inhaled steroids to control their symptoms, and some may also have inhalers that give a long-acting bronchodilator action.

Whichever type of treatment the patient has, they should all be instructed by a nurse who has training in respiratory disease (or a doctor) on how to recognise their symptoms and manage them quickly and effectively. Never underestimate the potential danger of an asthma attack. All patients should seek emergency help if their symptoms are getting worse as asthma can deteriorate very quickly.

Chronic obstructive pulmonary disease (COPD)

In 2022, 1.4 million people in the UK were diagnosed with COPD, making this the second most common lung disease after asthma. The prevalence increases with age, and 2% of the whole population (4.5% of people older than the age of 40) have been diagnosed with COPD (Asthma and Lung UK 2022). This figure may well underestimate the true figure, though, due to the prevalence of undiagnosed cases and this may lead to an under allocation of resources (Stone et al. 2023).

COPD is usually associated with smoking, and because smoking levels are much higher in some disadvantaged sectors of the community, these people tend to be disproportionately affected by COPD compared with the rest of the population. (ASH 2023).

COPD can also have occupational causes such as exposure to dust or toxins. A small percentage of people with the disease may have inherited a condition called alpha-1 antitrypsin deficiency, which results in destruction of the alveoli – the tiny air sacs at the end of the bronchioles.

So, what is it?

COPD is a term used to describe various conditions, including chronic bronchitis, **emphysema**, chronic obstructive airways disease and chronic airflow limitation. Patients with COPD experience progressive breathlessness, chronic productive cough and limited exercise capacity. This is caused by airflow obstruction that is not reversible in the way that asthma is. There is permanent damage to the airways, and treatment options are limited.

Managing COPD

Smoking cessation is the most important treatment, and it is never too late to stop, despite what the patient may think. If the disease is in the early stages and symptoms are mild, no other treatment may be needed. Even if the patient has been a heavy smoker for most of their life, stopping smoking can still slow down the progression of the disease.

Treatments for stable COPD include the following.

- **Bronchodilator** inhalers (e.g. salbutamol, terbutaline, salmeterol).
- **Antimuscarinic** inhalers (e.g. ipratropium, tiotropium).
- Steroid inhalers (e.g. beclometasone, fluticasone, budesonide).

- Combination inhalers.
- Bronchodilator tablets.
- **Mucolytic** medicines, which make the sputum less sticky and easier to cough up.

Treatments to manage exacerbations include the following.

- Steroid tablets to reduce the inflammation in the airways.
- Antibiotics.
- Admission to hospital.

Treatments for end-stage COPD include the following.

- **Domiciliary** oxygen – this can only be prescribed by a hospital specialist.
- **Palliative** care to keep the patient as comfortable as possible, including physiotherapy and rehabilitation.
- Exercise training.
- Support and advice.
- Medication for depression and anxiety may also be required.

The HCA role in caring for patients with COPD is an important one, and includes:

- promoting healthy living;
- monitoring bloods, blood pressure, lung function testing and pulse oximetry;
- encouraging influenza and pneumococcal vaccination;
- supporting patients and carers;
- referring patients with early signs or increasing problems;
- recognising and referring patients with associated depression and anxiety; and
- keeping up to date with current developments and guidelines.

LUNG FUNCTION TESTING

Peak flow recording

The peak flow measures the fastest rate of air blown out of the lungs in litres per minute. It can be used in the diagnosis and monitoring of asthma. Readings are dependent on the height, age and gender of the patient, and a normal range can vary by up to 100 litres per minute more or less than the predicted level. Charts with normal peak flow values are

Understanding lung function and disease

available online. Type 'peak expiratory flow rate – normal values' into your search engine.

Recording the peak flow measurement: the procedure

You can download the National Occupational Standard CHS19 *Undertake Routine Clinical Measurements* to use as a checklist for your competencies (Skills for Health 2021).

1. Check the patient's identity and obtain informed consent.
2. Decontaminate your hands.
3. The patient should be standing or sitting upright so that the lungs can fully expand.
4. Insert a disposable mouthpiece with a 'one-way' valve into the peak flow meter. Use the appropriate size mouthpiece according to the age of the patient.
5. Set the pointer on the meter to zero and ask the patient to hold the meter underneath so that their hands do not interfere with movement of the pointer.
6. The patient should then take a full breath in, seal their mouth around the mouthpiece, and blow hard and fast for 1–2 seconds.
7. Try to ensure that the patient remains upright when blowing. The natural tendency is to lean forward when blowing, but this will interfere with the lung expansion and deflation, and the reading will not be accurate.
8. Always repeat the process three times and record the best of the readings. It is often useful to demonstrate the procedure to the patient using your own mouthpiece.
9. Sometimes patients cannot perform this procedure properly; if this is the case, you must document this. If in doubt, seek advice from the nurse.
10. Document the measurement and report any low readings.

Spirometry

Asthma and COPD can be diagnosed by performing spirometry to measure how quickly and effectively the lungs can be emptied and filled. Measurements include the following.

- The amount of air the patient can blow out quickly and forcibly (i.e. the forced expiratory volume in one second, FEV1).

- The total amount blown out in one breath (i.e. forced vital capacity, FVC).
- FEV1/FVC (a low value indicates narrowed airways).
- The degree of reversibility following administration of a bronchodilator (e.g., salbutamol).

Age, height and gender will affect lung volumes.

COPD is categorised as mild, moderate or severe depending on the result, as follows.

- Mild (stage 1): FEV1 is at least 80% of the predicted value.
- Moderate (stage 2): FEV1 is 50–79% of the predicted value.
- Severe (stage 3): FEV1 is 30–49% of the predicted value.
- Very severe (stage 4): FEV1 is less than 30% of the predicted value.

Cleaning the equipment

Prior to the procedure, the equipment must be calibrated according to the manufacturer's instructions. Calibration may need to be done before every spirometry session and every four hours, or after every ten patients (whichever happens first). Results should be recorded in a calibration log. If the calibration shows any discrepancies, the equipment should be cleaned and rechecked. Do not continue with testing until the equipment has been successfully calibrated.

Cleaning should also be carried out in accordance with the manufacturer's instructions and local infection control policies. You should keep a cleaning log that must be signed and dated. Always use a one-way mouthpiece or bacterial filters.

Performing spirometry: the procedure

Please remember (as stated at the beginning of this chapter) that you should only perform lung function testing (including spirometry) if you have undergone an appropriate assessment and are able to demonstrate that you have achieved the standards established by the ARTP. This is because if the test is not performed to a high standard, there is a significant risk of incorrect diagnosis and potentially incorrect treatment resulting in harm to the patient (NHS England 2020).

Bearing this in mind, the following guidelines for performing spirometry are for general information only, and you should refer to your ARTP training notes for up-to-date information on how to perform the procedure accurately.

Understanding lung function and disease

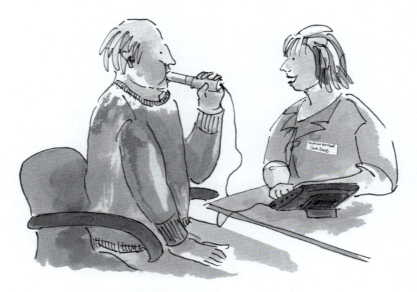

Figure 19.1 Performing spirometry

The patient should have been advised not to smoke for at least an hour before (preferably 24 hours if possible), not to have had a heavy meal for at least four hours, not to have had an alcoholic drink for at least four hours, not to have had any vigorous activity for 30 minutes and not to wear restrictive clothing. Any deviations from these requirements should be documented.

If the patient is attending for routine monitoring, they can have their inhalers as usual. If they are attending for baseline reversibility testing, they should have no short-acting bronchodilator for four hours, no long-acting bronchodilator for eight hours, and no sustained-release bronchodilators for 36 hours.

1. Check the patient's identity and obtain informed consent.
2. Decontaminate your hands before and after the procedure.
3. Check that there are no **contraindications** (see Box 19.2).
4. Make sure that they have an empty bladder!
5. Record age, gender and height.
6. The patient should be seated upright in a chair with arms. Both their feet should be flat on the floor.
7. Advise the patient to loosen any tight clothing and remove any false teeth if they are loose-fitting.
8. Perform the slow vital capacity before the forced vital capacity. This is done first because the airways are likely to collapse prematurely

when the patient with COPD tries to blow out hard. Place a nose clip on the patient or ask them to hold their nose. Ask the patient to breathe in as deeply as they can, place their lips around the mouthpiece to form a seal, and then blow out slowly and steadily for as long as they can. This is almost like sighing. Wait at least 30 seconds before repeating, and then repeat twice if possible, to ensure the results are consistent, accurate and reproducible.

9 Now perform the forced vital capacity. Remove the nose clip. Ask the patient to take a deep breath in, place their lips around the mouthpiece to form a seal, and then blow out forcibly and rapidly for as long as they can until they have no breath left to blow out. This should take from 6–15 seconds. Take a minimum of three readings if possible. Wait at least 30 seconds between each attempt. The best two readings should have the FVC within 100 ml of each other.

10 The patient may need encouragement to keep blowing until they cannot blow any more, and it is helpful to place a hand lightly on their shoulder to stop them from leaning forward. This is a normal response to get all the breath out, but by doing this they will inadvertently compress the lungs a little and render the result inaccurate.

11 Advise the patient not to cough or take another breath during the procedure, as this will invalidate the result. You can usually tell when this has happened, as there will be a characteristic step in the flow chart. Watch out for anything else that may interfere with the results, such as poor effort, leakage around the mouthpiece, a slow start or an abrupt stop. If any of these things happen, the results should be discarded and the test done again.

12 Stop the procedure if the patient feels unwell at all during the procedure and seek advice from the nurse or doctor. A maximum of eight blows is recommended. If the acceptability criteria are not achieved after this, the test should be stopped and rebooked for a later date if appropriate.

13 Record:

- FEV1 and the percentage of the predicted FEV1;
- FVC and the percentage of predicted FVC;
- peak flow (PEF); and
- FEV1/FVC.

REVERSIBILITY TESTING

This only needs to be done if there is doubt over the diagnosis and to identify asthma.

Understanding lung function and disease

1   The patient should be prescribed a bronchodilator inhaler (usually salbutamol).
2   Measure the FEV1.
3   The patient should then take four puffs of the inhaler via a large volume spacer.
4   After 15 minutes, remeasure the FEV1. If there is an increase of more than 12% from the baseline reading, this indicates reversible airflow obstruction and supports the diagnosis of asthma.

You should not administer salbutamol unless it has been prescribed for the individual patient or there is a patient-specific direction (PSD) for salbutamol in place for that patient (for more information about PSDs, see Chapter 20).

Box 19.1 Triggers for asthma

- Cigarette smoke (passive or active smoking).
- Cold air.
- Pollen.
- Dust.
- Dust mite faeces.
- Animal hair.
- Chemicals such as solder fumes, glues and aerosols.
- Respiratory infection.
- Stress/emotion.
- Exercise.
- Laughter.
- Some medications, such as beta blockers and non-steroidal anti-inflammatories.
- Mould.

Box 19.2 Contraindications to spirometry (*procedure should not be performed*)

- Previous problems when performing spirometry.
- Current active chest infection.
- Current acute illness or any communication issues that could interfere with the ability to perform the test properly.
- Patient has been coughing up blood.

- Suspected or active tuberculosis (TB).
- Unstable heart disease/angina.
- Recent **pneumothorax** (three months).
- Recent eye surgery.
- Recent abdominal or chest surgery (three months).
- Diagnosed **aneurysm** (thoracic, abdominal or cerebral).
- Refer to the registered nurse if the patient has ear problems, has a history of fainting, has a diagnosis of glaucoma or is pregnant.

Now try the following quiz. You can check back in the text for the answers

LUNG FUNCTION QUIZ

1. Why do we need oxygen?
2. What is the purpose of the alveolus?
3. What is meant by total lung capacity?
4. List three possible symptoms of asthma.
5. How many readings should you take when performing a peak flow rate?
6. What is the most common cause of COPD?
7. What does FEV1 stand for?
8. What does a low value of FEV1/FVC indicate?
9. Why should you perform a slow vital capacity before the forced vital capacity?
10. What should be in place before you administer salbutamol to the patient for reversibility testing?

Using a framework for reflection (see Chapter 2), try reflecting on a consultation when you performed lung function testing. How did it go, and what did you learn?

REFERENCES

Allen, M. (2023) *RightCare Asthma Scenario*. https://www.england.nhs.uk/wp-content/uploads/2023/02/Rightcare-Asthma-Scenario-feb-2023.pdf (accessed October 6, 2024).

Arshad, H., Karmaus, W., et al. (2012) The effect of parental allergy on childhood allergic diseases depends on the sex of the child. *Journal of Allergy and Clinical Immunology* 130(2): 427–434. https://www.

sciencedirect.com/science/article/abs/pii/S0091674912006112 (accessed October 6, 2024).

ASH (2023) *Smoking Statistics*. https://ash.org.uk/uploads/Smoking-Statistics-Fact-Sheet.pdf (accessed September 6, 2024).

Asthma and Lung UK (2022) *COPD in the UK: Delayed Diagnosis and Unequal Care*. https://www.asthmaandlung.org.uk/sites/default/files/2023–03/delayed-diagnosis-unequal-care-executive-summary.pdf (accessed November 4, 2024).

NHS England (2020) *Spirometry Commissioning Guidance*. https://www.england.nhs.uk/wp-content/uploads/2020/03/spirometry-commissioning-guidance.pdf (accessed October 6, 2024).

NICE (2017 updated 2021) *Asthma: Diagnosis, Monitoring and Chronic Asthma Management*. https://www.nice.org.uk/guidance/ng80 (accessed October 6, 2024).

NICE (2023 Revised 2024) *What is the Prevalence of Asthma?* https://cks.nice.org.uk/topics/asthma/background-information/prevalence (accessed October 6, 2024).

Skills for Health (2021) *CHS19 Undertake Routine Clinical Measurements*. https://tools.skillsforhealth.org.uk/competence-details/html/4371 (accessed September 13, 2024).

Stone, P., Osen, M., Ellis, A. et al. (2023) Prevalence of chronic obstructive pulmonary disease in England from 2000 to 2019. *International Journal of Chronic Obstructive Pulmonary Disease* 18: 1565–1574. https://pubmed.ncbi.nlm.nih.gov/37497381 (accessed October 6, 2024).

Thomas, M. (2018) *If, When and How to Use FeNO*. http://www.pulsetoday.co.uk/clinical/clinical-specialties/respiratory-/if-when-and-how-to-use-feno/20036595.article (accessed October 6, 2024).

Administering immunisations

20

Administering injections such as influenza, pneumococcal pneumonia, shingles and COVID-19 vaccines is something that HCAs have been doing successfully now for several years. However, it wasn't so many years ago that I attended a nursing conference when the first discussions about this task being delegated to HCAs were occurring, and there was uproar! Many nurses thought that in the absence of regulation and recognised HCA training, it was a step too far and was putting patient safety on the line. Now, of course, HCAs are routinely and safely administering the routine vaccines for adults, and some HCAs are giving vitamin B_{12}, vitamin D, heparin and insulin injections, as well as human papilloma virus (HPV) vaccines. What you do will depend very much on the area where you work and your local policy, but should also be dependent on you having the appropriate training and documentation in place such as the PSD (discussed later in this chapter). You must also be up to date with resuscitation training and anaphylaxis management.

This chapter will discuss the HCA role in giving those vaccinations that are covered by the National Minimum Standards and Core Curriculum for Immunisation Training of Healthcare Support Workers (PHE 2015). This publication is, of course, pre-pandemic and so does not include COVID-19 immunisations in its recommendations, but it is now widely accepted that these are suitable vaccines for the HCA to administer providing that they have had the appropriate training and are using a PSD.

There will be an overview of the diseases and the vaccines, but you will need to refer to *The Green Book: Immunisation Against Infectious Disease* for more detailed and current information (The Green Book 2013). All chapters are updated regularly as necessary. It is constantly referenced throughout this chapter because it is an essential source of information for all vaccinators.

Vitamin B_{12} (in the form of hydroxocobalamin) is an injection (but *not* an immunisation) that is routinely administered by HCAs in primary care, so there is information about this at the end of the chapter.

DOI: 10.4324/9781003460381-25

WHY DO WE NEED THE MINIMUM STANDARDS?

Immunisation programmes are one of the most successful public health measures to prevent disease, but it is essential to maintain public confidence in the programme to ensure its continued success. When confidence is dented, the uptake of vaccines goes down, with resulting peaks in disease levels. A good example of this is the measles epidemic that occurred following scare stories (based on discredited research) about the alleged adverse effects of the MMR (measles, mumps and rubella) vaccine. Vaccination levels went down and the number of measles and mumps cases rose dramatically, resulting in permanent injury and deaths (Pepys 2007; McIntyre and Leask 2008). More recently, outbreaks of measles have caused problems in areas where vaccination uptake is lower. During the COVID-19 pandemic, there were several myths circulating on social media regarding the vaccination which have since been disproven (ZOE.com 2023), but such misinformation has the power to derail an effective vaccination programme – and it cannot be ignored. Always take your information from good sources and have the facts on hand for when your patients ask you questions about the vaccines. If you don't feel confident to discuss the evidence with them, then refer them to the nurse or doctor. We must always make sure that when people are given an injection, they can have confidence in the vaccination and in the person administering it.

The National Minimum Standards (PHE 2015) were developed to support and facilitate high-quality, safe delivery of the influenza, pneumococcal and shingles vaccination programme. Although Public Health England (PHE) no longer exists, the standards for healthcare support workers (HCSWs) are still entirely relevant and are outlined in Box 20.1 (with the COVID-19 immunisation included).

Box 20.1 Standards for immunisation training of HCSWs

- HCSWs must have completed relevant training and been assessed as competent.
- The practitioner who delegates the role of immunisation must be on a relevant professional register and must ensure that the HCSW has met the necessary standards of competency.
- Any HCSW who immunises should receive specific training and annual updates.
- The training content should include specific core areas of knowledge.

- The recommended duration of training is a minimum of two days, with annual half-day updates.
- HCSWs with a role in immunisation should have access to all updates of national influenza, COVID-19, shingles and pneumococcal vaccination policy, as well as *The Green Book: Immunisation Against Infectious Disease* (2013).
- HCSWs actively involved in immunisation services must have an identified supervisor who should be a registered, appropriately trained, experienced and knowledgeable practitioner.
- Staff training at all levels should be included in a regular audit of the immunisation service.

How can you keep updated?

Once you agree to get involved in giving injections, you must make sure you keep updated, as guidelines and vaccines are constantly changing. There are several ways to do this, including the following.

1 Attend the annual flu and COVID-19 updates that should be provided locally. Sometimes these may be in the form of online learning.
2 Look up *The Green Book* (2013) online and keep it handy. It is an indispensable reference for all types of immunisation and includes chapters on every aspect. The individual chapters are regularly updated to reflect all current policy regarding specific vaccines and injection techniques.
3 Subscribe to vaccine updates. Type 'gov.uk' into your search engine and look for *vaccine updates*. If you subscribe to these, you will get a monthly newsletter with up-to-the-minute information on any changes in policy, programmes, etc. Not all the information will be relevant to you (as with *The Green Book*), but it is easy to sift out what you need.

WHAT IS A VACCINATION, AND HOW DOES IT WORK?

Immunity can be inborn or acquired.

- *Inborn immunity* is basically the immunity you are born with. It includes physical barriers, such as skin and mucous membranes, and chemical barriers, such as the acid in your stomach. Inborn immunity is useful for disposing of some pathogens before they can cause us any harm, but it is not as effective as acquired immunity.

- *Acquired immunity* can be passive or active.

  - *Passive immunity* occurs – as the name suggests – 'passively', and involves the transfer of antibodies across the placenta or via the breast milk. It can also be provided by an injection of immunoglobulin. This type of immunity is useful, but the antibodies transferred in this way will only last for a few days or weeks, and so only provide short-term protection. They do not stimulate the body to produce its own antibodies, so there is no 'immunological memory'. Consequently, if the body is exposed to the disease again in the future, it will have no protection against it.
  - *Active immunity* is long-lasting and occurs when the body is exposed to the actual disease or to a vaccine that mimics the disease. The invading **antigen** (e.g. bacteria or virus) stimulates the body's immune system into producing chemicals called antibodies that neutralise the antigen. This is the best type of immunity because the antibodies will remain in the system as memory cells, and if the body is exposed to the same disease again in the future, the antibodies can be reactivated to provide protection.

Vaccines contain weakened (also referred to as attenuated) or inactivated parts of the disease-causing organism. They trick the body into thinking it has been exposed to the actual disease without producing the unpleasant effects. The immune system produces antibodies in response, and the immunological memory will then 'recognise' the antigen that causes the disease, so if the body is exposed to it again, it will produce the appropriate antibodies as and when required.

Different types of vaccine

- *Live attenuated vaccines*: These vaccines are made of weakened or altered disease-causing organisms. They cannot cause the actual illness, but because the organism has not been killed, they can still cause unpleasant effects in somebody with an impaired immunity. Examples of these types of vaccines include the influenza nasal spray and shingles vaccines.
- *Inactivated/killed organisms or viruses*: With these vaccines, the organism has been completely disabled, so it will never cause the disease it is designed to protect against. An example of an inactivated vaccine is the seasonal injectable influenza vaccination for adults.

- *Segments of the pathogen*: These will not cause the disease they are designed to prevent, but will still be able to trick the immune system into thinking it has been invaded by the whole pathogen. An example of this type of vaccine is the pneumococcal pneumonia vaccine.
- *mRNA vaccines*: Messenger ribonucleic acid (mRNA) provides a way of using the instructions in our genes (deoxyribonucleic acid, or DNA) to make specific proteins in our cells. In vaccines, this results in the production of a harmless piece of protein identical to one found in a specific bacterium or virus. The immune system recognises this protein as a 'foreign body' and produces antibodies to attack it if encountered again in the form of the actual virus or bacterium. The COVID-19 vaccine is an example of this.
- *Recombinant vaccines:* These are made through genetic engineering whereby the gene that creates the protein for a virus or bacteria is placed inside the genes of another cell. When that cell reproduces, the vaccine proteins produced are recognised by the immune system. An example of this type of vaccine is Shingrix®.

Vaccination will protect the individual who receives it, and that person is then less likely to pass infection to others. This reduces the infection risk for unvaccinated people, so it protects them, as well. This is called *herd immunity* or *population immunity*. If vaccination coverage is high enough, this may eventually lead to the eradication of a specific disease (as has happened with smallpox).

Storage of vaccines: the cold chain

All vaccines should be kept at 2–8°C from the moment they are manufactured to the moment they are administered. This is an essential feature of a vaccination programme because vaccines will lose **efficacy** if they are exposed to inappropriate temperatures for too long, so this can be very wasteful and expensive for the NHS, and the vaccine may no longer provide the required immune response. NHS England (2021) has issued a list of recommendations to ensure maintenance of the cold chain (see Box 20.2).

Box 20.2 Recommendations for correct storage of vaccines

- Nominated cold chain lead should be responsible for receiving vaccines. Before signing for delivery, vaccines must be checked to ensure that there is no damage to packaging and no leakage. Record the type, brand, quantity, batch number, expiry date,

> date and time of receipt, running total of vaccines and signature of person receiving delivery. Vaccines must be refrigerated immediately on receipt in original packaging, maintaining the cold chain at all stages.
>
> - Store vaccines in a lockable validated vaccine fridge at 2–8°C (a mid-range of 5°C is good practice), with space for the air to circulate. The fridge must only be used for vaccines and medicines.
> - Rotate all stock so that those with the shortest expiry date are used first. Avoid over-ordering.
> - Use switchless sockets to avoid accidental disconnection.
> - *Read* and *record* fridge temperature at the same time every working day and sign the record sheet (minimum and maximum temperatures). *Reset* thermometer after each reading. *React* if temperature falls outside 2–8°C.
> - Use a validated medical-grade cool box for storing vaccines during transfer of stock.

LEGAL ISSUES FOR HCAS ADMINISTERING INJECTIONS

HCAs should only administer *injectable* medication to people *aged 16 or older* and can also administer *intranasal* vaccines to children aged 2–18 (for more on consent and record-keeping, see Chapter 7).

The patient-specific direction

This is the tricky bit! Every year, HCAs are signed up for immunisation courses in the mistaken belief that they will then be able to administer the injections in the same way as registered nurses. It comes as a bit of a blow to some students (and managers) to realise that this isn't the case. While registered nurses can work under legal frameworks called patient group directions (PGDs), there is a more stringent legal framework called the patient-specific direction (PSD) that must be in place before unregistered health workers can administer an injection. When I used to deliver updates every year, I was constantly amazed at how many HCAs have (unknowingly) acted illegally, because they have been giving injections without a PSD in place. It is essential that you understand what the PSD is to ensure patient safety and to make sure that you are acting within the law and are covered by your insurance provider.

So, what is the difference between the PSD and the PGD?

The PSD is a written (manual or electronic) instruction, signed by a doctor, dentist or non-medical prescriber for medicine to be supplied and/or administered to a named patient after the prescriber has assessed the patient on an individual basis.

The PSD can also be an instruction to administer a medicine to a list of named patients whereby each patient on the list has been individually assessed by the prescriber. The prescriber must have knowledge of the patient's health and be satisfied that the medicine serves the individual needs of each patient on that list (CQC 2022a, 2022b).

It is good practice for the PSD to include the surgery (or workplace) details, the prescriber's name and qualification, the HCA's name and the name, dose, route and frequency of the injection. The PSD should also specify a start and finish date.

The prescriber has a duty of care and is legally and professionally accountable for delegating the task to the HCA, so they must be completely sure that the HCA has had the appropriate training as outlined in the National Minimum Standards (PHE 2015) and is competent to administer injections.

Just to be clear, a PSD:

- is *not* the same as an FP10 (traditional prescription);
- is *not* the same as a simple signature on the bottom of a list of names;
- is *not* a verbal instruction;
- is *not* the same as a PGD template that has been renamed a 'PSD'; and
- is *not* the same as a generic instruction to be applied to any patient who fits the eligibility criteria and who happens to attend on a specific day.

Patient group directions

These are suitable for registered and specified staff, and comprise written instructions for the supply or administration of medicines to groups of patients who may not have been individually identified before presenting for treatment. It is the responsibility of the person administering the medicine to assess the patient beforehand, and the PGD is therefore *not* suitable for HCAs working at levels 3 or 4.

Having read this, you might be feeling as if it is hardly worth taking on this task when the patient must be assessed before you can give the injection anyway. But the good news is that it *is* possible, and many thousands of HCAs are now giving injections safely and legally. It just takes a little bit of forward thinking and preparation.

An example of a PSD template is provided in Box 20.3, but there are others available online. Just be careful that the one you use adheres to the legal requirements!

Box 20.3 Example template for a patient-specific direction (attach this to the clinic list of patients or scan on to individual patient's notes)

Administration of inactivated influenza vaccination by an HCA/AP

Name of practice: ....

Address: ....

Name of vaccine (please print): ....

Dose: ....

Route: ....

This PSD is valid from: .... to .... [insert dates as applicable]

Name of prescribing practitioner: ....

Status: ....

Signature: .... Date: ....

Name of supervising practitioner: ....

Status: ....

Signature: .... Date: ....

Name of HCA 1 (print): ....

Signature: .... Date: ....

Name of HCA 2 (print): ....

Signature: .... Date: ....

THE DISEASES AND THE VACCINES

Influenza

Influenza is an acute viral infection of the respiratory tract. There are three types of influenza virus, known as A, B and C, with A and B responsible for most clinical illness. Virus A causes outbreaks and is the usual cause of epidemics. Virus B causes less severe disease and smaller outbreaks. Illness due to virus C is not as common and tends to be milder.

These viruses are subject to slight changes every year, and this is known as antigenic drift. Periodically, a major change in the virus occurs, and this is called antigenic shift. This usually results in a new subtype of virus that is likely to cause epidemics or even **pandemics**.

Symptoms of flu can be mild or severe, but it is not the same as a bad cold, and it usually has a longer recovery period.

ACTIVITY

Flu is a more severe illness than a cold and tends to come on more quickly.

How many symptoms of flu can you think of?

Check your answers in Box 20.7, as well as in Figure 20.1.

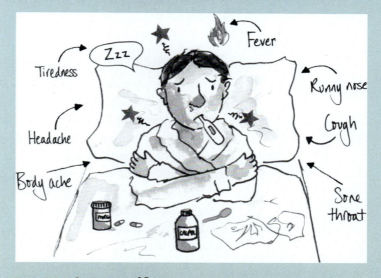

Figure 20.1 Symptoms of flu

It is highly infectious and spreads rapidly, especially in closed communities. The virus is spread in respiratory droplets when a person coughs or sneezes, or via contaminated surfaces such as door handles. Some research has also shown that flu can be passed between people by simply breathing (University of Maryland 2018).

The flu virus can live for many hours on hard surfaces, so the advice from the Department of Health and Social Care (2013) was to catch coughs and sneezes in a paper tissue and then wash hands to kill the germs – 'Catch It, Bin It, Kill It!' – a slogan that is still widely used.

An outbreak of flu can have a big impact, especially on vulnerable members of society such as the very young or very old, pregnant women, morbidly obese, people with immunodeficiency or no spleen, and those who have a chronic disease. Each year, thousands of people die from complications after catching the flu, but figures vary from year to year.

During the 2023–2024 season in England, deaths due to influenza were estimated to be quite low at 2,776 compared to 15,465 in the previous season (UK Health Security Agency 2024a).

Complications include things such as:

- bronchitis;
- secondary bacterial pneumonia;
- otitis media (middle ear infection);
- meningitis; and
- encephalitis.

The flu vaccine

Flu viruses are constantly changing, so the vaccine composition is reviewed annually and updated. In February every year, the WHO assesses the flu strains that are most likely to be circulating during the following winter in the northern hemisphere. Depending on which ones are most likely to spread and cause illness, the WHO then recommends which three or four flu strains (usually two A viruses and one or two B viruses) should be used in the vaccines for the next season. It is not easy to predict exactly which viruses are going to cause problems, and sometimes it goes wrong, such as happened in the 2014–2015 season when the A (H3N2) virus produced a subtype after the vaccine strain had been selected, so the vaccine was not as effective.

The flu vaccines used in the past have not been very effective at all in the older age groups (over 75), and in 2018, a flu vaccine was developed that is more effective against the H3N2 strain in this age group. The Joint Committee on Vaccination and Immunisation advised the use of the adjuvanted trivalent (containing three virus types, i.e., two A and one B) influenza vaccine (aTIV) in the over-65 age group. In 2020, a quadrivalent formulation of the adjuvanted vaccine (aQIV) was also granted licensure for the same age group. An **adjuvant** is a substance added to the vaccine that improves efficacy.

Since December 2018, a high dose trivalent vaccine (TIV-HD) also became available and is licensed for the older age group. This vaccine contains four times the antigen content of standard TIV and produces a stronger immune response (The Green Book 2013, Chapter 19 updated November 2023).

A universal flu vaccine is also being developed, which may mean that people will only need one or two flu vaccines in their life, but this is not available yet (University of Oxford 2017).

If this is used in the future, it will put an end to flu clinics as we now know them!

There are two types of flu vaccine:

- the *injectable* flu vaccine for adults (and children younger than 2); and
- the *intranasal* flu vaccine for children from the age of 2 up to the age of 18 (live attenuated influenza vaccine, or LAIV).

Most of the flu viruses to be used for the vaccine have historically been grown on hens' eggs and then deactivated for the injectable vaccine or weakened in the intranasal LAIV, then purified before being made into the vaccine. Contrary to popular belief, they cannot cause flu in the vaccinated person. However, patients who have an egg allergy must be offered vaccines that are egg-free or that have a low ovalbumin (egg protein) content.

According to data from surveillance of the UK 2018–2019 season, both the aTIV and TIV-HD appear to be more cost-effective than unadjuvanted vaccines grown on hens' eggs in the older age group (The Green Book 2013, Chapter 19 updated November 2023) and with the increasing prevalence of cell cultured vaccines such as the QIVc, the issue of allergy associated with vaccines cultured on hens' eggs may soon become a problem of the past.

The vaccine is always aimed at the most vulnerable members in the population, as outlined previously. However, eligibility criteria will vary from year to year, so you will need to check the annual flu plan for England (or equivalent for Wales, Scotland and Northern Ireland), which is usually available from May onwards.

Injectable inactivated flu vaccine

This can be either trivalent or quadrivalent. It is usually supplied as a single dose of 0.5 ml suspension in a prefilled syringe with an integral needle. It should be administered intramuscularly into the deltoid muscle in the upper arm or the vastus lateralis muscle in the **anterolateral** aspect of the thigh.

Individuals who have a bleeding disorder should usually have their injections via the subcutaneous route when possible, although at least one of the adjuvanted trivalent vaccines can only be given via the intramuscular route, so always first check the information leaflet (summary of product characteristics, or SPC).

Contraindications

Do not give to anyone who has had a confirmed anaphylactic reaction to a previous dose or to any component of the vaccine.

Precautions

Postpone if the patient is acutely unwell with pyrexia.

Adverse reactions are common, but usually disappear within one to two days. They include things such as:

- pain, swelling or redness at the injection site;
- low-grade flu-like symptoms; and
- a small painless nodule at the injection site.

Live attenuated influenza vaccine (LAIV)

This is a quadrivalent vaccine and is supplied as a suspension in a special applicator that is designed for intranasal use only. In the UK, it is only to be used for children aged from 2–18. The dose is 0.2 ml, and the applicator is designed to allow a dose of 0.1 ml per nostril. Current guidelines advise two doses for children aged 2–9 who have never had the vaccine before and who are in clinical risk groups. The two doses should be given at least four weeks apart (The Green Book 2013, Chapter 19 updated November 2023). If the LAIV is not available for the second dose, then the injectable quadrivalent vaccine may be used, but must then be given by the registered nurse.

The vaccine contains gelatine from pigs, which may make it unacceptable for some religious groups and vegetarians.

Contraindications (more details are available in The Green Book)

The LAIV is a *live vaccine*, which means that the virus used in the vaccine has been weakened but not killed. This will not be an issue for most children who have a healthy immune system, but may be for those who have any form of impaired immunity. For this reason, the list of contraindications is longer than for the inactivated injection. *It is important to remember this!*

Do not give to anyone who:

- has had a confirmed anaphylactic reaction to a previous dose or component of the vaccine;

- has clinical severe immunodeficiency;
- has severe asthma or is actively wheezing, or has been prescribed oral steroids in the last 14 days for respiratory disease;
- is on salicylates; or
- is known to be pregnant.

Precautions

Postpone the vaccine if the child is heavily congested or unwell with a fever.

When you are unsure about anything, always check with the nurse or doctor before giving the vaccine. You might think that if the patient is covered by a PSD, then they have been assessed as fit to receive the vaccine by the prescriber (and hopefully they will have been), but remember that *you* are accountable for giving this vaccine, and even if they are covered by the PSD, you must *not* give the vaccine if they have a contraindication or you suspect that they might have.

Adverse reactions are common, but usually settle quickly.

Common

- nasal congestion or runny nose;
- reduced appetite;
- weakness; and
- headache.

Less common

- pyrexia/malaise;
- rash; and
- nosebleed.

Pneumococcal disease

Pneumococcal disease is a term used to describe infections caused by the bacterium *Streptococcus pneumoniae* (also called pneumococcus). More than 90 different types have been identified. The bacteria can spread into the sinuses to cause sinusitis or into the middle ear cavity to cause otitis media (middle ear infection). It may also affect the lungs to cause pneumonia, and can cause systemic (invasive) infections such as bacteraemic pneumonia, bacteraemia and meningitis.

It is spread by respiratory droplets, but unlike with flu transmission, it usually requires either frequent or close contact. It can occur at any time of the year, but peaks in the winter months.

It is a major cause of morbidity and mortality, particularly affecting the very young, the elderly and those with impaired immunity. Recurrent infections can occur in association with skull defects, cerebrospinal fluid leaks, cochlear implants and skull fractures (The Green Book 2013, Chapter 25 updated August 2023).

Pneumococcal vaccine for adults

Pneumococcal polysaccharide vaccine (PPV23) is the vaccine that is most commonly given to adults, and it contains 23 of the different types of bacteria that account for approximately 96% of serious infection in the UK. It is supplied as a single dose of 0.5 ml and administered intramuscularly into the deltoid muscle of the upper arm or vastus lateralis muscle in the anterolateral thigh. It can also be given subcutaneously if the patient has a bleeding disorder.

For most people, one dose will be enough, but in some groups, such as those with splenic dysfunction or severe kidney disease, the **antibody** levels decline more rapidly. For this reason, these groups will be offered the vaccine every five years.

The vaccine is aimed at vulnerable groups, such as the elderly and the very young, those with chronic disease, and those with a problem that may make them more prone to problems with the bacteria (e.g., those people with a skull fracture and those who have had cochlear implants). Current eligibility can be checked in The Green Book (2013, Chapter 25 updated August 2023).

Contraindications

Confirmed anaphylaxis to a previous dose or any component of the vaccine.

Precautions

Postpone if the patient is acutely unwell with pyrexia. Pregnant and breastfeeding women who need this vaccination should be referred to the registered nurse.

Adverse reactions are not common, but may include things such as:

- mild soreness and induration at the site of injection lasting one to three days;
- low-grade fever; and
- severe systemic reactions (rare).

Herpes zoster (shingles)

Shingles is also known as zoster or herpes zoster, and it is caused by the same virus that is responsible for chickenpox (the varicella zoster virus)

Most of us will have had chickenpox (or been exposed to it) as a child. The problem with this virus is that even after we have recovered from the acute illness, the virus stays in the body. It lies dormant in the nerve cells and can reactivate at a later stage, usually when the immune system is weakened. Anyone who has had chickenpox can get shingles.

The incidence and severity tends to increase with age. You have about a 1 in 4 chance of developing shingles at some time in your life.

When the virus is reactivated, it travels from the clusters of nerve cell bodies (ganglia) in the spinal nerve to the area supplied by that nerve in the skin. The nerves supply various areas called dermatomes, and the shingles rash will typically affect very specific areas on one or the other side of the body (see Figure 20.2).

While the virus is travelling along the nerve, it causes symptoms such as pain, tingling or itching and numbness. There may also be generalised malaise, headache and fever. When it reaches the skin, the virus produces a blistering rash, usually with intense pain and itching. The rash will typically last for 2–4 weeks (see Box 20.4)

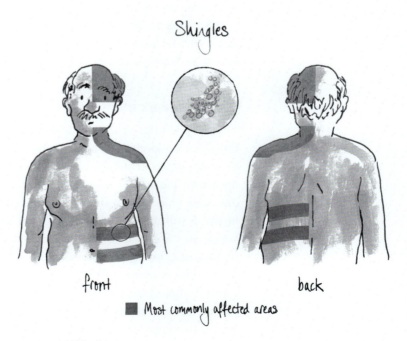

Figure 20.2 Shingles

Box 20.4 Symptoms of shingles

- Abnormal skin sensations or pain in the affected area.
- Headache, photophobia, malaise and occasionally fever may occur before the rash appears.
- Within days or weeks, a unilateral (one-sided) vesicular rash (fluid-filled blisters) appears in a dermatomal distribution.
- The affected area may be intensely painful, with tingling, pricking or numbness and intense itching.
- The rash typically lasts between two and four weeks.

You cannot catch shingles from somebody else with shingles, but you can catch chickenpox from shingles if the lesions are still blistering and uncovered and you have close contact with that person (assuming you haven't had chickenpox before).

Complications of shingles

Post-herpetic neuralgia (PHN) is nerve pain that persists in the affected area, typically lasting for 3–6 months, and sometimes longer. The severity of the pain varies, and it may be triggered by stimulation, such as touch or wind on the face.

Other complications will depend on the area affected, and may include things such as facial palsy, eye problems (e.g. keratitis, retinitis and corneal ulceration), pneumonia, hepatitis and encephalitis.

Shingles vaccine

The complications of shingles often result in hospitalisation and sometimes death, especially in older people. Treatments for shingles tend to have side effects or simply don't work very well. The vaccine was developed with the aim of reducing the incidence and severity of shingles disease in older adults, among whom the risk and severity of disease is higher. It will also save a huge amount of money for the NHS because of saved hospital days, doctor appointments and prescriptions. Based on the findings of a cost-effectiveness analysis, the Joint Committee on Vaccination and Immunisation (JCVI) recommended a universal routine herpes zoster (shingles) vaccination programme using Zostavax®, a live, attenuated virus, for adults aged 70–79 years. This older age group was considered likely to have the most benefit from the vaccination. In the first five years of the programme in England, it was estimated that approximately

45,000 GP appointments and nearly 2,000 hospitalisations were averted because of vaccination with Zostavax® (Green Book 2013, Chapter 28a updated April 2024).

From September 2023, Zostavax® was replaced by Shingrix® in the routine immunisation programme. Shingrix® is a non-live recombinant vaccine, available as a white powder to be reconstituted with diluent (after which it becomes a colourless to pale brown liquid) and is injected as a suspension. Inspect the reconstituted vaccine for any particles or unusual appearance; if either is observed, do not administer the vaccine. It must be used promptly after reconstitution or stored in a refrigerator (2–8°C) or discarded if not used within 6 hours.

Adults should receive two doses of 0.5 ml of Shingrix® with an interval of 6–12 months in England, Wales and Northern Ireland (eight weeks to six months in Scotland). For severely immunosuppressed adults, the second dose should be given between eight weeks and six months after the first dose to give the individual protection more quickly. The injection should be given intramuscularly into the deltoid region of the upper arm. It should not be given subcutaneously.

Contraindications

- Confirmed anaphylactic reaction to a previous dose or any component of the vaccine.
- Current acute episode of shingles.

Precautions

- Care is required where the individual has thrombocytopenia or any coagulation disorder as bleeding may occur following IM injection. These patients should be booked in with the nurse.

COVID-19

COVID-19 is a disease of the respiratory system caused by the SARS-CoV-2 virus, which is primarily spread through respiratory droplets and aerosols and from direct person-to-person contact. Symptoms commonly include headache, cough, fatigue and myalgia. Severe infection can result in pneumonia, acute respiratory distress syndrome, multiple organ failure and death.

I'm sure you can still remember those depressing death tolls read out on the news every day during 2020–2021 when the pandemic was at its height. New strains of the virus are emerging fairly regularly but so far have not been associated with any major increases in incidence. In the UK, 4.5% of patients report variable long-term symptoms affecting physical and mental health and this is currently an area of ongoing study (Green Book 2013, Chapter 14a updated September 2024)

Children with the infection generally remain asymptomatic or develop mild disease only with upper respiratory tract symptoms, and most children in the UK now have natural immunity to SARS-CoV-2 due to natural infection in the younger age groups.

There are many different vaccines available for use in the UK now, and you should check *The Green Book* online (Green Book 2013) and your vaccine updates from gov.uk for the most current information

B$_{12}$ DEFICIENCY

We all need vitamin B$_{12}$ to help us create red blood cells and to keep our nervous system healthy. It is also needed to absorb folic acid and release energy, and it is essential to lower the levels of a chemical called homocysteine. High levels of this chemical are associated with heart disease and stroke.

If we are lacking in B$_{12}$, we will eventually be unable to produce enough red blood cells, and will therefore be unable to carry enough oxygen around the body, resulting in **anaemia**, but don't get confused – this type of anaemia has nothing to do with iron deficiency! There are different types of anaemia with different causes, but ultimately they all interfere with our ability to carry oxygen, and so we exhibit the same sorts of symptoms.

> Anaemia occurs when the body is unable to transport oxygen efficiently, usually because there are fewer red blood cells than normal or there is not enough haemoglobin in the red cells.

ACTIVITY

How many symptoms of anaemia can you think of?

Check your answers against the list in Box 20.5.

Because B$_{12}$ is also important for a properly functioning nervous system, a deficiency can also result in neurological symptoms such as tingling fingers and toes, confusion, memory loss, and muscle weakness.

Vitamin B$_{12}$ is a water-soluble vitamin that is naturally present in some foods such as meat, poultry and dairy produce. It is added to other foods and is available as a dietary supplement and a prescription medication. Vitamin B$_{12}$ is also known as the 'extrinsic factor' because it comes from outside the body. We produce a chemical in the parietal cells of the stomach lining called the 'intrinsic factor'. This enhances the absorption of vitamin B_{12}, which then occurs further down in the gut at the end of the small intestine.

Box 20.5 Symptoms of anaemia

- Extreme tiredness.
- Lack of energy.
- Breathlessness.
- Feeling faint.
- Dizziness.
- Palpitations.
- Headaches.
- Pale skin.
- Tinnitus.
- Loss of appetite and weight loss.

Anaemia caused by B_{12} and folate deficiency may also cause further symptoms, including:

- pale yellow tinge to the skin;
- sore red tongue (glossitis);
- mouth ulcers;
- pins and needles in the hands and feet;
- disturbed vision;
- irritability;
- reduced sense of taste;
- changes in movement;
- muscle weakness;
- changes in thoughts, feelings and behaviour;
- decline in mental abilities; and
- diarrhoea.

(NHS Choices 2023)

Causes of B_{12} deficiency

- *Pernicious anaemia* is the most common cause of B_{12} deficiency. It is an autoimmune disorder (when the body attacks itself) because the immune system makes antibodies that act against the parietal cells in the stomach or against the intrinsic factor produced by those cells.

This means that the patient is unable to absorb enough B_{12}. Incidentally (if you take blood), this is the reason why you may be asked to do a blood sample for 'intrinsic factor antibodies' or 'parietal cell antibodies'. It is a check for pernicious anaemia.

- *Inflammatory bowel disease* (e.g. Crohn's disease or ulcerative colitis). This interferes with absorption of B_{12} lower down in the intestine.
- *Some diets*, such as a vegan diet, because B_{12} is not found in vegetables or fruit, but it is available in yeast extract, fortified cereals, soya milk and soya products.
- *Excessive alcohol* because this causes inflammation or atrophy of the stomach lining, and may therefore interfere with the effect of the intrinsic factor.
- *Some drugs*, such as metformin. A large percentage of patients who are on long-term metformin will develop B_{12} deficiency. This is an important point to remember because metformin is given to patients who have diabetes. These patients may often have a complication of their diabetes called peripheral neuropathy where the nerves are damaged. This results in tingling, pain or numbness of the toes, but this is also a symptom of severe B_{12} deficiency. It is quite possible that such symptoms will be attributed to the diabetes when in fact they may be due to B_{12} deficiency caused by their metformin. Such neurological damage is irreversible, and the importance of detecting this deficiency early is now well recognised. It is therefore important to monitor those diabetic patients on long-term metformin for B_{12} levels to check for B_{12} deficiency (Chapman et al. 2016; MHRA 2022).

B_{12} injection

When the patient has B_{12} deficiency because they cannot absorb vitamin B_{12} from the gut, they will usually be prescribed replacement therapy with injectable hydroxocobalamin, which is a form of B_{12}. The injection is a clear red liquid presented as 1 mg/ml (or 1,000 mcg/ml) in a glass ampoule. It must be stored at a temperature of less than 25°C and it should be protected from light, in its box.

Open a pre-injection swab and use the empty packet as a cover for the top of the ampoule. You can then break the top of the ampoule into the cover.

Breaking the neck of a glass ampoule and drawing up the fluid can be tricky and takes practice. I hope you'll be shown how to do this during your immunisation training, but failing that, ask your nurse to show you the first time. There are also plenty of YouTube video tutorials – watch a good one before you try it, and remember to protect your hands from glass fragments! If you do it properly, there should be a clean break with minimal glass fragments. It would be very embarrassing to be standing there with bloodied hands in front of your patient after breaking a glass ampoule incorrectly!

Hydroxocobalamin is given intramuscularly into the deltoid muscle of the upper outer arm, or into the vastus lateralis in the anterolateral thigh. It can be given subcutaneously if the patient has a bleeding disorder.

Most patients will have a significant reduction in their levels of B_{12} by the time they are diagnosed, so they need a large dose initially to boost their levels. This is called the loading dose, and usually comprises six injections, one every 2–4 days over two weeks. There is no reason why the HCA cannot give the loading doses, providing the PSD is specific about the dose and the dates that the injections should be given. After the loading doses, the usual maintenance dose is one injection every 12 weeks, but if the patient has developed neurological symptoms, they may be offered it at eight weekly intervals.

When designing a PSD for a hydroxocobalamin injection, it makes sense to prepare one that can then be inserted into the patient's notes and used each time the patient presents. There is no need to make out a new one each time, as it is the same medication and same dose. It is useful to state in the PSD that the patient should be given the injection every 12 weeks (or every eight weeks), *or three days either side of the due date*. This allows a little flexibility for those patients who are unable to attend on a specific day.

Contraindications

Hypersensitivity to any ingredient (but this is rare).
Adverse reactions are rare, but may include symptoms such as a rash, nausea, diarrhoea, pain at injection site, headache or irregular heartbeat.

GIVING AN INJECTION: THE PROCEDURE

You can download the Royal College of Nursing document *Immunisation Knowledge and Skills Competence Assessment Tool*, third edition, which provides an excellent guide to the type of record you should complete as evidence of your competence in giving an immunisation (RCN 2022), although please note that some sections are not applicable to the HCA role in immunisation.

There is also a specific assessment tool for COVID-19 (UK Health Security Agency 2024b)

You must attend an appropriate training course and have written evidence of your competence before giving injections.

1 Prepare your patient (see Box 20.6).
2 Make sure the patient is sitting down (preferably) with their arm relaxed by their side or in their lap. The injection site should be fully exposed. If you are injecting into the deltoid muscle, make sure the upper arm is adequately exposed. If the sleeve is rolled up, it should not be too tight as this works as a tourniquet and may make the patient bleed. Only clean the skin with soap and water if the skin is visibly dirty. There is no need to use alcohol swabs.
3 Decontaminate your hands. There is no need to wear gloves.
4 Prepare the equipment. Some flu vaccinations are prefilled with an integral needle, but for other injections, you may need to prepare the syringe, needle and injection.
5 Check the vaccine/injection to make sure you have the correct product and the correct dose, and that it is not past the expiry date. If you are giving a vaccine, check that the cold chain has been maintained.
6 Examine the colour and composition of the vaccine/injection and ensure it conforms with the SPC. If you are unsure about this, it can usually be found in a leaflet inside the box.
7 If the injection is prefilled (e.g. inactivated flu vaccine), there is not usually any need to expel the air from the syringe (PHE 2014).
8 Injections that are supplied as suspensions (e.g. inactivated influenza) will need to be shaken before administration.

Box 20.6 Preparing the patient

- Check patient identity.
- Check that the PSD is in place for that patient.
- Explain the procedure and make sure your patient (or person with parental responsibility, if giving LAIV to a patient younger than 16) gives informed consent. Include information about advantages, disadvantages, possible side effects and their management in your explanation, and offer a patient advice leaflet.
- Ask the following questions:

  - Do you feel unwell today?
  - Have you had (name of injection/vaccine) before?

Administering immunisations

- Have you had any reaction to a vaccination/medication before?
- Do you have an egg allergy? (prior to giving inactivated flu vaccine only)
- Are you pregnant or breastfeeding? (prior to giving LAIV, shingles or pneumococcal vaccine)
- Do you have lowered immunity due to disease or treatment? (prior to giving LAIV or shingles vaccine)
- Do you have a bleeding disorder? (If the answer to this is 'Yes', it is suggested that injections should be given by the deep subcutaneous route to reduce the bleeding risk [Specialist Pharmacy Service 2023], but this may not be necessary and may be outside of the product licence. Therefore in this instance, seek advice from the doctor or nurse).

Intramuscular (IM) injection technique

IM injections are usually given with a blue needle (25 mm long, 23 gauge) for a person of average build. Larger patients with more subcutaneous fat will need a longer needle (green, 38 mm long) to ensure the medication is given into the muscle and not into the subcutaneous layer. An individual assessment must be made, and if you are unsure, check with the registered nurse first.

- *Locate the injection site* over the deltoid muscle by drawing an imaginary line two fingers' breadth below the acromion process (shoulder tip). The injection should be given into an imaginary triangle whose base is formed by the line and whose apex will be in line with the axilla. This ensures that the injection is given into the belly of the muscle for optimum absorption and effect (see Figure 20.3).
- *Stretch the skin* over the injection site between the thumb and forefinger of your non-dominant hand. With your dominant hand, hold the syringe near the tip (like a pencil or dart) and insert the needle at a 90-degree angle to the skin, all the way in (see Figure 20.6). Make sure the hand holding the syringe is somehow in contact with the patient's arm, either by extending your little finger or by resting the edge of your little finger on the skin. This keeps you in control of the syringe and needle in case the patient moves (see Figure 20.4). Push the plunger in steadily (at about 1 ml per second) until all the medication has been given. Take the needle straight out and have cotton wool ready in case there is a spot of blood, but don't rub the area.

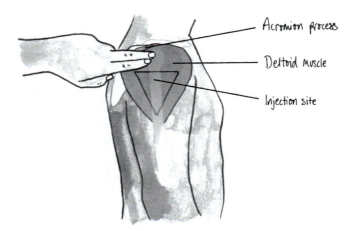

Figure 20.3 Intramuscular injection site

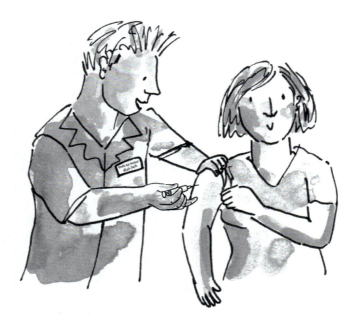

Figure 20.4 Giving an intramuscular injection

- *Some local policies are promoting the Z-track technique.* To do this, you need to locate the area as before, but instead of stretching the skin, push the skin to the side of the site before inserting the needle at 90 degrees. Push the plunger of the syringe steadily to administer the vaccine. Leave in position for 10 seconds, then remove the needle and allow the skin to move back into place. This makes a seal in the muscle and prevents leakage of the medication into the surrounding tissue.

Subcutaneous (SC) injection technique

SC injections are usually given with an orange needle (16 mm long, 25 gauge).

- *Locate the injection site*, which is usually on the upper outer arm (see Figure 20.5).
- *Bunch the skin* over the area using the thumb and forefinger of the non-dominant hand. With your dominant hand, hold the syringe comfortably so that you can insert the needle at a 45-degree angle to the skin, all the way in (see Figure 20.6). Try to keep the hand that is holding the syringe in contact with the patient's arm so if they move, you move with them! Push the plunger in steadily until all the medication has been given. Take the needle straight out and have cotton wool ready in case there is a spot of blood, but don't rub the area.

9 Dispose of the needle and syringe immediately into a sharps bin, which should be close at hand.
10 Apply a small plaster or cotton wool and tape if necessary (but remember to check for allergies first).
11 Observe the patient for signs of immediate adverse reaction.

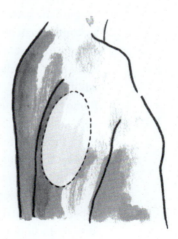

Preferred site for SC injection is upper outer arm

Figure 20.5 Subcutaneous injection site

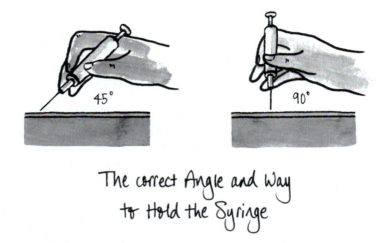

Figure 20.6 Needle angles for subcutaneous and intramuscular injections

12 Decontaminate your hands.
13 Document the procedure, including the following information:

- consent obtained;
- no contraindications;
- vaccine name, batch number, dose, route, site, expiry date;
- any problems; and
- name of immuniser and date of administration.

GIVING AN INTRANASAL VACCINATION (LAIV): THE PROCEDURE

1 Prepare the patient (see Box 20.6).
2 Decontaminate your hands.
3 Make sure the child is sitting comfortably with their head slightly tilted back. Toddlers should be held securely on the accompanying adult's lap.
4 Remove the rubber tip protector. Do *not* remove the dose divider clip.
5 Place the tip just inside the nostril, and with a single rapid motion, depress the plunger until the dose divider prevents you from going any further. This will deliver 0.1 ml into the nostril. Use a rapid motion when depressing the plunger to achieve a fine mist, which is better absorbed by the nasal mucosa. If you push the plunger too slowly, the liquid comes out in a dribble, and is likely to run out of the nose and not be absorbed as effectively.

Administering immunisations

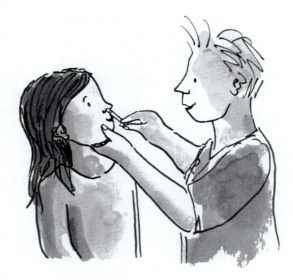

Figure 20.7 Giving an intranasal vaccine

6 Pinch and remove the dose divider clip and administer the remaining dose in the other nostril in the same way as before.
7 The patient should breathe normally and not sniff.
8 If their nose runs or they sneeze following the procedure, reassure them that the vaccine will still be effective, and they do not need to have it again.
9 Observe the patient for signs of immediate adverse reaction.
10 Decontaminate your hands.
11 Document the procedure as for the IM and SC techniques.

Box 20.7 Symptoms of flu

- Sudden onset of fever (less likely with a simple cold) and chills or rigours.
- Headache.
- Myalgia (aching muscles).
- Extreme fatigue.
- Dry cough.
- Sneezing and sore throat (sometimes).
- Nasal congestion.
- May be vomiting and diarrhoea (e.g. as in swine flu).
- Recovery in seven days – sometimes longer.
- May require hospitalisation.

Now try the following quiz. You can check back in the text for the answers.

VACCINATION AND B12 QUIZ

1. What is the difference between passive and active immunity?
2. What is the difference between a live vaccine and an inactivated vaccine?
3. What temperature should vaccines be stored at?
4. What legal framework must be in place before an HCA can administer an injection?
5. What age group is the LAIV used for in the UK?
6. When giving the intranasal vaccine, should the plunger be pressed rapidly or slowly?
7. Is the Shingrix® shingles vaccine live or inactivated?
8. Why do we need vitamin B_{12}?
9. Should the skin be stretched or bunched for an intramuscular injection?
10. What is the angle of insertion for the needle when giving an intramuscular injection?

TIME TO REFLECT

Using a framework for reflection (see Chapter 2), try reflecting on a consultation when you watched or gave a vaccination or other injection.
How did it go, and what did you learn?

REFERENCES

Care Quality Commission [CQC] (2022a) *GP Mythbuster 19: Patient Group Directions (PGDs)/Patient Specific Directions (PSDs)*. https://www.cqc.org.uk/guidance-providers/gps/gp-mythbusters/gp-mythbuster-19-patient-group-directions-pgdspatient-specific-directions (accessed July 5, 2024).

Care Quality Commission [CQC] (2022b). *HealthCare Assistants in General Practice*. https://www.cqc.org.uk/guidance-providers/gps/gp-mythbusters/gp-mythbuster-57-health-care-assistants-general-practice (accessed August 16, 2024).

Chapman, L., Darling, A., and Brown, J. (2016) Association between metformin and vitamin B12 deficiency in patients with type 2 diabetes: A systematic review and meta-analysis. *Diabetes & Metabolism* 42(5): 316–327. https://www.ncbi.nlm.nih.gov/pubmed/27130885 (accessed October 14, 2024).

Department of Health and Social Care (2013) *'Catch it. Bin it. Kill it': Campaign to Help Reduce Flu Infections.* https://www.gov.uk/government/news/catch-it-bin-it-kill-it-campaign-to-help-reduce-flu-infections (accessed October 14, 2024).

McIntyre, P., and Leask, J. (2008). *Improving Uptake of MMR Vaccine.* https://www.ncbi.nlm.nih.gov/pmc/articles/PMC2287215/ (accessed October 6, 2024).

Medicines and Healthcare Products Regulatory Agency [MHRA] (2022) *Metformin and Reduced Vitamin B12 Levels: New Advice for Monitoring Patients at Risk.* https://www.gov.uk/drug-safety-update/metformin-and-reduced-vitamin-b12-levels-new-advice-for-monitoring-patients-at-risk (accessed October 14, 2024).

NHS Choices (2023) *Symptoms. Vitamin B12 or Folate Deficiency Anaemia.* https://www.nhs.uk/conditions/vitamin-b12-or-folate-deficiency-anaemia/symptoms (accessed November 7, 2024).

NHS England (2021) *Vaccine Storage and Handling – Cold Chain Policy.* https://www.england.nhs.uk/east-of-england/wp-content/uploads/sites/47/2022/07/East-Cold-Chain-Policy-April-2021-v5–6.pdf (accessed October 9, 2024).

Pepys, M. (2007) Science and serendipity. *Clinical Medicine* 7(6): 562–578. https://www.ncbi.nlm.nih.gov/pubmed/18193704 (accessed October 6, 2024).

PHE (2014) *Air Bubbles in Syringes. Vaccine Update Issue 222.* https://assets.publishing.service.gov.uk/government/uploads/system/uploads/attachment_data/file/383514/VU_222_Nov_DEC_2014_09_Accessible.pdf (accessed October 14, 2024).

PHE (2015) *Core Curriculum for Immunisation Training of Healthcare Support Workers.* https://assets.publishing.service.gov.uk/media/5a806c8740f0b62305b8b12d/HCSW_Training_Standards_September_2015.pdf (accessed October 6, 2024).

RCN (2022) *Immunisation Knowledge and Skills Assessment Tool.* https://www.rcn.org.uk/Professional-Development/publications/immunisation-knowledge-and-skills-competence-assessment-tool-uk-pub-010–074 (accessed October 14, 2024).

Specialist Pharmacy Service SPS (2023) *Using Intramuscular Injections in People on Oral Anti-Coagulants.* https://www.sps.nhs.uk/articles/using-intramuscular-injections-in-people-on-oral-anticoagulants (accessed October 14, 2024).

The Green Book (2013) *Immunisation Against Infectious Disease.* https://www.gov.uk/government/collections/immunisation-against-infectious-disease-the-green-book (accessed November 25, 2024/November 4, 2024).

UK Health Security Agency (2024a) *Surveillance of Influenza and Other Seasonal Respiratory Viruses in the UK, Winter 2023 to 2024.* https://www.gov.uk/government/statistics/surveillance-of-influenza-and-other-seasonal-respiratory-viruses-in-the-uk-winter-2023-to-2024 (accessed October 14, 2024).

UK Health Security Agency (2024b) *COVID-19 Vaccinator Competency Assessment Tool.* https://assets.publishing.service.gov.uk/media/66fe9f333b919067bb482be0/COVID-19-vaccinator-competency-assessment-tool-September–2024.pdf (accessed October 14, 2024).

University of Maryland (2018) *Flu May Be Spread Just by Breathing: Coughing and Sneezing Not Required for Transmission.* www.sciencedaily.com/releases/2018/01/180118142611.htm (accessed October 14, 2024).

University of Oxford (2017) *World-First Trial for Universal Flu Vaccine.* http://www.ox.ac.uk/news/2017-10-03-world-first-trial-universal-flu-vaccine (accessed October 12, 2024).

ZOE.com (2023) *Are Sharks Being Killed for COVID Vaccines? Does the Vaccine Contain Monkey Cells? And Will it Alter Your Genes? We Tackle the Most Common COVID-19 Vaccine Myths.* https://zoe.com/learn/covid-vaccines-myths (accessed October 9, 2024).

Ear irrigation

21

In recent years, HCAs and APs have been taking on more complex tasks such as ear irrigation, although, unfortunately, it is not usually performed in general practice any longer – and because of this, I was unsure about including this chapter in the third edition of this book. However, it is one of those services that I truly believe to be essential for some patients, and I hope it will one day be fully reinstated as a free service in primary care. Furthermore I am aware of some APs setting up their own private ear irrigation services – and for this reason, I decided to keep this chapter in the book. Removal of earwax is one of those rare things you can do for your patient that can provide instant relief when their hearing has been compromised by a build-up of wax, but unfortunately it is a task that has provoked much controversy over the years. This is largely because the old method of syringing the ears using a metal syringe often resulted in problems afterwards, such as perforation or infection (Aung and Mullet 2002). This in turn resulted in litigation in many cases. By comparison, removal of wax using an electronic irrigator is a very safe procedure, providing that it is done in accordance with the guidelines. However, although irrigation is relatively safe, there are risks associated with it, as with any procedure. Bearing this in mind, before agreeing to examine a patient's ear or irrigating it, you must complete a recognised ear irrigation course, such as the one offered by the Rotherham Ear Care Centre and Audiology Service (2024). These courses are available all over the UK and are delivered by trainers who are licensed to the Ear Care Centre. Other courses are available, but always make sure the course providers have a good reputation and can offer accredited training.

A good background understanding of ear anatomy and physiology, as well as a thorough practical training in the procedure, is essential if this task is to be carried out safely. This chapter will provide the background knowledge required and will describe the procedure in line with the Rotherham Ear Care Centre guidelines.

DOI: 10.4324/9781003460381-26

EAR ANATOMY AND THE HEARING PROCESS

The ear is divided into three parts, usually described as the outer, middle and inner ear (see Figure 21.1).

The outer ear

The outer ear is made up of the pinna (see Figure 21.2) and the external auditory meatus (ear canal). The pinna is the external structure, and is designed to collect and direct the sound waves into the ear canal. The ear canal is a skin-lined channel ending at the outer surface of the tympanic membrane (TM, or eardrum).

The middle ear

The middle ear is the area behind the eardrum where three little bones are located. These tiny bones, known by their Latin names as the malleus, the incus and the stapes, are collectively called the ossicles. These bones have joints between them in the same way as other groups of bones do, and they are the only bones in your body that should not grow from the moment you are born to the moment you die!

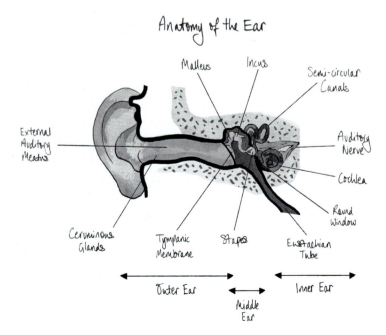

Figure 21.1 Ear anatomy

Ear irrigation

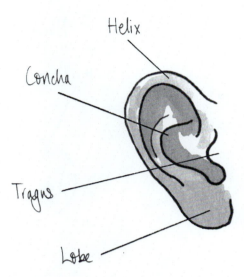

Figure 21.2 External ear

Sound waves are channelled through the pinna into the ear canal, and they hit the eardrum, making it vibrate. This vibration is transmitted through the ossicles into the inner ear.

The malleus is the bone that sits against the eardrum from behind and gives it the characteristic shape. It is the features of this bone that you look for during otoscopy. Remember, the eardrum is made up of a soft part – pars flaccida (seen above the short process of the malleus) and the taut part, which is stretched tightly over the long process of the malleus (also called the handle of the malleus), making it transparent and shiny – the pars tensa (seen below the short process of the malleus). The light reflex is created where the long process of the malleus creates a crease in the pars tensa, which picks up and reflects the light from the otoscope (see Figure 21.3).

The inner ear

The inner ear consists of the cochlea (organ of hearing) and the semicircular canals (organ of balance).

The cochlea is a coiled structure with inner channels that are filled with fluid. Vibrations are transmitted from the ossicles, through the oval window (a membrane covered opening underneath the stapes) into the fluid-filled channels, where they create ripples. The ripples pass over tiny hairs called cilia located deep within the cochlea, and the subsequent movement of the cilia sends a signal via the auditory nerve to the brain, where it

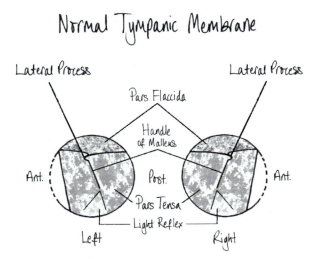

Figure 21.3 Eardrum features

is then interpreted as noise. The brain is usually able to determine where the noise is coming from and what is causing it. This whole process is very complex and delicate. If the sound waves are created by a very loud noise, then their amplitude will be greater, and this will cause bigger vibrations and bigger ripples. When the ripples become very big, instead of wafting the cilia gently, they will flatten them all, like a field of corn in a hurricane. Not all the cilia will recover from this, and those that do will recover at different rates. This can result in abnormal signals being sent to the brain, creating buzzing or ringing in the ears and a reduction in hearing for a while. Think of the last time you went to a music gig – what happened when you came out? You were probably shouting at each other for a while until your hearing recovered! If our ears are constantly exposed to loud noise, then early onset deafness is inevitable as more and more of those cilia are flattened and unable to recover.

The semicircular canals operate in a similar way, except that the signal sent back to the brain is interpreted as a sense of position instead of noise.

WAX

Many patients seem to think that wax is dirty and should be cleaned out of the ear regardless of whether it is causing a problem or not. Wax is actually very important for protection, lubrication and slowing down the growth of bacteria. It is made up of cerumen (a sweat-like substance), sebum (an oily substance), dead skin cells and debris. The composition of wax will vary from individual to individual, depending on age, diet and the environment. The ceruminous glands, where the cerumen is produced, are located just inside the ear canal. This is a fact worth pointing out to your patients when the wax is seen pushed up against their eardrum, usually because of poking cotton buds or other small items in the ear!

Sometimes it may be necessary to remove wax by irrigation, but this should always be a last resort because putting water inside the ear canal increases the risk of infection.

ACTIVITY

Consider what wax is made up of and then list as many factors as you can think of that may make the patient more susceptible to increased or impacted earwax.

Check your answers in Box 21.1.

Softening the wax

Olive oil drops at room temperature are the cheapest and most suitable way of softening the wax. The patient should be instructed to instil the drops every morning and evening for 3–5 days. They should lie on the unaffected side for ten minutes after instilling the drops and avoid the use of cotton wool in the ear. An olive oil ear spray is available on prescription and can be bought over the counter, and this may be very useful for your elderly patients who live alone and find it difficult to instil the drops.

It is always worth advising patients who have a frequent build-up of wax in their ears to instil olive oil drops regularly (once or twice a week), as this is sometimes all that is needed to soften the wax and facilitate the natural cleaning process of the ear without the need for irrigation.

Sodium bicarbonate can also be used (Patient.info 2022), but this can have a drying effect, especially in the elderly who tend to have a drier and thinner meatal skin.

Box 21.1 Factors that may increase wax accumulation

- Fatty diet/high cholesterol.
- Excessive sweating.
- Narrow ear canals – Down's syndrome patients tend to have narrower ear canals, which makes them more prone to problems with earwax (National Deaf Children's Society 2018).
- Noisy or dusty environment.
- Age.
- Genetics.

EAR IRRIGATION: THE PROCEDURE

Only those patients who have had the procedure done previously with no complications are suitable for the HCA to irrigate. Patients must be assessed by the doctor or nurse first to determine the presence of wax and their suitability for irrigation. If most of the eardrum is visible, then irrigation will not normally be necessary. The only exception to this will be if the patient is to have a hearing aid fitted, in which case the ear canal must be completely clear.

The procedure outlined in Box 21.2 is adapted from the Rotherham NHS Foundation Trust (2022).

- Assemble the equipment (see Box 21.2).

Box 21.2 Equipment for ear irrigation

- Electronic irrigator (Projet or Propulse current model).
- Disposable jet tips.
- Warm water (37°C).
- Otoscope and disposable speculae (with good batteries).
- Headlight (with good batteries).
- Single-use Noots tank or equivalent. A disposable plastic bag liner in a metal Noots tank is a cheaper alternative to the disposable cardboard variety and takes up less space.
- Single-use Jobson Horne Probe or equivalent.
- Cotton wool.
- Disposable waterproof cape.
- Tissues.
- Disposable gloves.
- Receiver for dirty cotton wool, etc.

- Check patient identity and obtain verbal informed consent. As part of this process, you should advise the patient of the possible risks, including the small risk of perforation and infection.
- Check for any contraindications or precautions (see Box 21.3).

Box 21.3 Ear irrigation: contraindications and precautions

Contraindications to irrigation

Do *not* irrigate the ear. Refer the patient back to the doctor.

- Never had the procedure done before.
- Previous complications following the procedure.

- Current perforation or history of mucus discharge from the ear in the last year.
- History of middle ear infection within the last six weeks (as there may be a perforation following production of infected mucus in the middle ear).
- Any ear surgery apart from grommets that have extruded 18 months previously.
- Outer ear infection (otitis externa) with pain.

Precautions

Check with the nurse or doctor for advice before proceeding.

- Healed perforation. The eardrum is not as strong and may re-perforate.
- Cleft palate (repaired or not). If there is an existing perforation as well, there is a risk of water being directed into the middle ear.
- Dizziness. Irrigation may make this worse.
- Tinnitus. Irrigation may make this worse.
- On oral anticoagulants. The ear canal is more likely to bleed.

- Decontaminate your hands.
- *Examine the ear* while sitting at the same height as the patient. Look around the pinna and check the surrounding scalp for any skin lesions, signs of previous surgery, infection or any other abnormalities.
- Examine *inside the ear canal* using an otoscope (preferably one with a white halogen fibre-optic light) fitted with the largest speculum that will fit comfortably into the ear canal. Straighten out the ear canal by *gently* grasping the cartilaginous part of the pinna and pulling upwards and outwards. Hold the otoscope like a pen or dart and rest your little finger on the patient's cheek while you insert the speculum into the ear canal (see Figure 21.4). Use the right hand to view the right ear and the left hand to view the left ear if you feel you can do this safely. If the wax is obscuring the eardrum and is soft enough, proceed with irrigation.
- Protect the patient with a waterproof cape.
- Put the headlight on.
- Put on the gloves. Earwax is a body fluid, and there is a small risk of contamination with hepatitis B (Kalcioglu et al. 2004).
- Explain the procedure to your patient and ask them to indicate if they have any pain or dizziness during the irrigation, in which case the

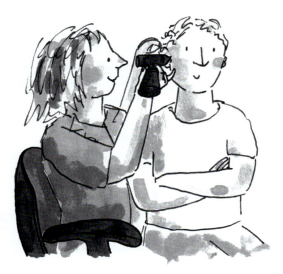

Figure 21.4 Using the otoscope safely

procedure should be stopped immediately and the patient referred to the nurse or doctor.
- Sit at the same height as the patient.
- Run the water through the tubing to expel any trapped cold water. This also helps the patient get used to the noise of the irrigator.
- Ask the patient to hold the Noots tank under their ear.
- Run a few drops of the water on to the patient's earlobe to check if the temperature is comfortable for them.
- Direct the headlight at the ear and – while gently lifting the ear upwards and outwards to straighten the ear canal – insert the jet tip just inside the ear, directing it towards the back of the head. If you imagine the eardrum like a clock face, the water stream should be directed at 11 o'clock for the right ear and 1 o'clock for the left ear (see Figure 21.5).
- Starting with minimum pressure, operate the foot pedal to direct a steady stream of water into the ear canal until the wax comes out. Keep the jet tip in the same position and avoid twisting it, as this may cause trauma to the ear canal.
- If no wax comes out after a few minutes, increase the pressure to medium. Check frequently with the otoscope to see if the wax is moving and to make sure there is no inflammation or bleeding in the ear canal, in which case the procedure should be stopped.
- Continue until the ear is clear and the eardrum visible or until one tank of water has been used. Use no more than one tank per ear. If you are unsuccessful at this stage, the patient should be advised to continue

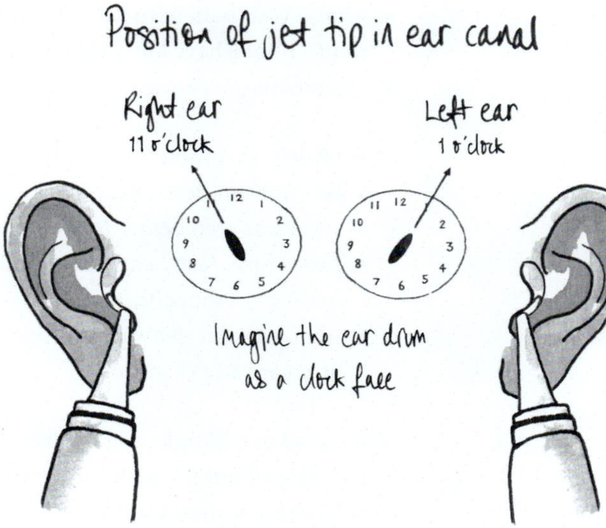

Ear irrigation

Position of jet tip in ear canal

Right ear
11 o'clock

Left ear
1 o'clock

Imagine the ear drum
as a clock face

Figure 21.5 Positioning the jet tip in the ear canal

with olive oil for a few more days before any further attempts are made to irrigate.

- When the irrigation is completed and the wax has been removed (or even if it has been unsuccessful), dry the ear canal carefully. Stagnation of water and abrasions sustained during the procedure will predispose to infection, so it is essential that dry mopping is performed properly. Ask the patient to tip their head to one side to allow the water to drain as much as possible. Then use cotton wool wrapped securely around the tip of the Jobson Horne Probe or carbon curette, and – with your headlight shining on the ear – insert the cotton wool-covered probe into the ear canal. Mop the skin of the ear canal, gently moving around the canal in a clockwise direction. Personally, I think good-quality cotton buds can also be used for this, and may well be a cheaper option instead of single-use probes or curettes, but please avoid giving patients the impression that it is OK for *them* to use cotton buds! (Use of cotton buds for drying the ear canal is advice based on the author's personal opinion, and is not included in the Rotherham Ear Care Centre guidelines.) The ear canal is only about 2.4 cm long, so keep your fingers near the tip of the probe to avoid putting it in too far, and always use a headlight so that you can visualise the tip.
- Examine the ear canal again using the otoscope and check that the eardrum is intact with normal features (see Figure 21.3).
- Remove your gloves and decontaminate your hands.

- Advise your patient to keep the ear dry for the next 24–48 hours and to return if they have any problems or concerns following the procedure.
- Document the process, including information as follows:

  - informed consent obtained;
  - no contraindications;
  - what was seen before (e.g. soft wax obscuring eardrum);
  - procedure (e.g. wax successfully or unsuccessfully irrigated, ear canal dry mopped);
  - what was seen afterwards (e.g. eardrum intact with normal features); and
  - aftercare advice given.

- Dispose of equipment in line with local policy.
- Decontaminate irrigator according to manufacturer's instructions or follow the Rotherham Ear Care Guidance document (see Box 21.4).

Tips

1   If the wax is proving stubborn to remove, ask the patient to open and close their mouth a few times. Jaw movement helps to dislodge wax, and this might be all that is needed.
2   If you're still having trouble, move on to the other ear (assuming the patient needs both ears irrigating) and then come back to the first ear. Sometimes the water left in the ear will act as a softener and the wax will come out easily after a few minutes. If only one ear is to be irrigated, ask the patient to sit out in the waiting room for ten minutes while you see to another patient and then try again.
3   If your patient starts to cough during the procedure, it is a good idea to stop. Coughing may indicate stimulation of the auricular branch of the vagus nerve that runs along the floor of the ear canal. The vagus nerve is responsible for controlling the heart rate and the BP, and if stimulated the heart rate and BP may drop suddenly, causing a vasovagal syncope (or faint). It is not worth continuing with irrigation in this case, as the risk of harm to the patient outweighs the benefits.

Box 21.4 Decontaminating the electronic irrigator

> Follow the manufacturer's instructions for the machine you are using. These may vary slightly from those given here.
> *Always wear appropriate PPE – such as gloves, apron and goggles – and only perform decontamination in a well-ventilated room.* This is because the solution used for decontamination (sodium dichloroisocyanurate,

NaDCC) is very toxic and can cause skin irritation and respiratory problems if inhaled.

The aim of the decontamination process is to clean out the stagnant water and solid particles from the tubing, and it should be carried out before every clinic when there are patients attending for ear irrigation. You should also decontaminate the equipment at the end of a busy clinic.

1 Discard the jet tip and dispose in the clinical waste.
2 Fill the tank with NaDCC solution made up as per manufacturer's instructions. Tablets such as Presept, Klorsept and Chlor-clean are suitable for this.
3 Flush the solution through to the end of the tubing and then leave for ten minutes (no longer).
4 Empty the tank and fill with fresh water. Flush the fresh water through the tubing until the tank is empty.
5 Dry carefully and store the machine in a cupboard until next required.

A bit about gadgets

Patients will often use all manner of gadgets to try to remove wax from their ears, and may well ask your advice about them, so it's good to have an idea of what is out there.

Try typing 'home earwax removal' into images on your search engine and I think you will be amazed and horrified at what is available for people to buy and stick into their ears! Basically, we should be discouraging people from putting 'anything smaller than their elbow' into their ear when they are unable to see what they are doing. This is unsafe practice, and is likely to lead to impaction of wax or infection in some patients.

Hopi candling is an alternative therapy that may be useful as a relaxation therapy, but it should not be used at home alone and it does not remove earwax (see Figure 21.6).

The Hopi candle is a fabric candle soaked in beeswax that is put into the ear while the other end is burnt down. The theory is that burning the candle softens the wax and creates a vacuum that sucks it out. This simply isn't true, and scientific evidence has clearly refuted this claim (Ernst 2004). At the end of the treatment, the client may be shown the 'earwax' along with other dirt and impurities that appear to be collected inside the remnants of the candle. This is simply the remnants of the burnt cotton and beeswax, and is *not* earwax! In fact, some patients who had no earwax to start with were found to have residues of candle wax in their ears following the procedure!

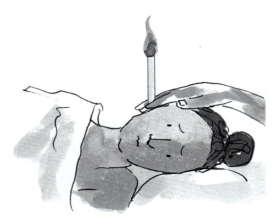

Figure 21.6 Hopi candling – not for wax removal

Quite apart from the fact that this practice does not remove earwax, it is intrinsically dangerous, and there have been many ear injuries associated with candling. So, while it may be used under supervision (and with great care) as an alternative therapy for relaxation, you should not be recommending this to your patients as a method of earwax removal (Rafferty et al. 2007).

Now try the following quiz. You can check back in the text for the answers.

EAR IRRIGATION QUIZ

1. Name the three bones found in the middle ear.
2. What are the two parts of the eardrum called?
3. The inner ear comprises the cochlea and the semicircular canals. Which of these is the organ of hearing?
4. What should be used to soften earwax, and for how long should it be used?
5. Why should you wear a headlight and sit at the same height as the patient when irrigating their ear?
6. Why might the patient cough when you are irrigating their ear?
7. What should you do following irrigation, regardless of if the procedure is successful or not, to reduce the risk of infection?
8. What will you do if the patient answers 'Yes' to any of the precautions?
9. What advice should you give your patient following the procedure?
10. Why is it important to decontaminate the irrigator in a ventilated room?

TIME TO REFLECT

Using a framework for reflection (see Chapter 2), try reflecting on a consultation when you watched or performed an ear irrigation.

How did it go, and what did you learn?

Remember, nobody died of earwax unless they didn't hear the bus coming!

REFERENCES

Aung, T., and Mullet, G. (2002) Removal of ear wax. *BMJ* 325: 27. https://www.bmj.com/content/325/7354/27 (accessed October 12, 2024).

Ernst, E. (2004) Ear candles: A triumph of ignorance over science. *The Journal of Laryngology and Otology* 118(1). https://www.ncbi.nlm.nih.gov/pubmed/14979962 (accessed October 14, 2024).

Kalcioglu, M., Durmaz, R., Ozturan, O. et al. (2004) Does cerumen have a risk for transmission of hepatitis B? *Laryngoscope* 114(3): 577–580. https://www.ncbi.nlm.nih.gov/pubmed/15091238 (accessed October 14, 2024).

National Deaf Children's Society (2018) *Down's Syndrome and Childhood Deafness*. https://ndcs.org.uk/family_support/childhood_deafness/causes_of_deafness/downs_syndrome.html (accessed November 7, 2024).

Patient.info (2022) *Sodium Bicarbonate Ear Drops*. https://patient.info/medicine/sodium-bicarbonate-ear-drops (accessed October 14, 2024).

Rafferty, J., Tsikoudas, A., and Davis, B.C. (2007) Ear candling. Should general practitioners recommend it? *Canadian Family Physician* 53(12): 2121–2122. https://www.ncbi.nlm.nih.gov/pmc/articles/PMC2231549 (accessed October 14, 2024).

Rotherham Ear Care Centre and Audiology Service (2024) *Home Page*. https://www.earcarecentre.com/professionals/training (accessed October 12, 2024).

Rotherham NHS Foundation Trust (2022) *Guideline for Ear Irrigation*. https://www.earcarecentre.com/uploadedFiles/Pages/Health_Professionals/Protocols/Ear%20irrigation%20guidelines%202022.pdf (accessed October 12, 2024).

Index

12-lead ECG 141–142, 145

ability 23–24
abuse 66–70
Access to Health Records Act (1990) 53
accountability 23–24, 66; *see also* delegation
acquired immunity 226
active listening 36
adjuvant 232
adrenal insufficiency 116
advice 74–75
agendas 40
aggression 48
alcohol 76, 78, 80, 242
alcoholism 111, 170
alginates 198
alveoli 137, 210, 213
Alzheimer's disease 42
ambulatory blood pressure monitoring (ABPM) 126
amputation 177, 181
anaemia 156, 205, 240, 241
anaerobic bacteria 198
anaphylactic reactions 234, 239
aneurysm 220
angina 128, 139, 220
anorexia 158, 170
antibiotics 92, 93, 197
antibodies 226, 227, 236, 241, 242
anticoagulants 150
antigen 226
antimicrobial dressings 197
antimuscarinic inhalers 213
ANTT *see* aseptic non-touch technique
anxiety: communication with patients 39–40; COPD 214; ECG procedure 143; physical activity 84; pulse rate 126; warning of risk 58
appearance 36, 38–39
aprons 92, 262
apyrexial 121
arrhythmia 116
arteries: atherosclerosis 181; blood pressure 125–126; foot assessment 184; heart anatomy 135–137; heart contraction 138;

heart disease 139; pulmonary 137; venepuncture 155
arterioles 137
arthropathy 180
asepsis 202
aseptic non-touch technique (ANTT) 98–99, 193, 201–202
assertiveness 40, 47–49
assistant practitioner (AP) 5–8, 9
associate practitioner *see* assistant practitioner (AP)
Association for Respiratory Technology and Physiology (ARTP) 209, 216
asthma 210–213, 215, 218–219
atherosclerosis 125, 181
atrial fibrillation (AF) 117, 121, 128, 140, 161
auscultatory method 128–129
authority 23, 24
autoimmune disease 178
axilla 122
Ayling Inquiry (2004) 101–102, 104

B_{12} deficiency 240–243
bacteria 92, 93, 196, 226, 227, 235, 236, 256
Baker, R. 101
best interests 47, 60
Bichard, Sir Michael 65–66
bile 157, 171
bilirubin 171
bleeding disorders 233, 236, 243, 245
blood circulation 121
blood clots 150, 157, 158
blood glucose *see* glucose
blood pressure 5–6, 33, 40, 125–132
blood taking *see* capillary blood testing; venepuncture
blood tests 54, 58, 149–164
body language 36, 42, 45
body mass index (BMI) 81, 111–113
body posture 37
body surface thermometers 122
bone disease 158
bradycardia 116
breast examinations 17, 18, 106–107
breathing 119–120, 141, 209–210, 211; *see also* lungs
brief intervention advice 74

British and Irish Hypertension Society (BIHS) 127
British Heart Foundation 29, 74, 127
British Hypertension Society 29
British Thoracic Society 30
broken record technique 49–50
bronchitis 213, 232
bronchodilator inhalers 212, 213, 216, 217, 219
bronchus 210
bullying 68
bundle of His 138

cadoxemer iodine 200
calcium 84, 158, 159, 194
Caldicott Report (1997) 55
cancer 77, 79, 82, 141, 156, 158
capacity 58, 60–61
capillaries 137, 210; foot assessment 184–185; skin anatomy 194; wound healing 195
capillary blood testing 161–163
carbohydrates 77, 79
carbon dioxide 119, 120, 137, 206, 209, 210
cardiac arrest 139
Care Certificate 7, 9
care plans 193, 197
Care Quality Commission (CQC) 29
catheters 125
cellulitis 92
chain of infection 93–94
chaperoning 18, 20, 101–107
Charcot foot 180–181, 183
chest pain 142
chickenpox 237–238
children: BMI 111; consent 59–60; DBS checks 104; immunisation 60, 228, 233–235, 240; physical activity 83
chloride 157
cholesterol 160: capillary blood testing 161, 163; earwax accumulation 157; healthy eating 76, 77; high blood pressure 132; physical activity 84
chronic obstructive pulmonary disease (COPD) 120, 156, 205, 213–216, 218
circulatory system 136–137

clinical guidelines *see* protocols
clotting process 149–150, 156
Code of Conduct for Healthcare Support Workers 20
codes of conduct 7, 21, 91
communication: avoiding interruptions and distractions 40; avoiding medical terminology 40; avoiding overfamiliarity 41; benefits 35; definition 35–36; fear, pain, anxiety and fatigue 39–40; language and cultural differences 40; methods 36; mismatched agendas 40; non-verbal communication 37–39; overcoming barriers to 39–41; personality clashes 40; with a person with dementia 44–46; practical difficulties 39; verbal communication 37
community-acquired infection (CAI) 92
competence 24, 25, 47, 67, 75, 150, 193, 244
compliance 35
Computer Misuse Act (1990) 53
concordance 35
confidentiality 50, 53–57
connective tissue 194
consent 57–61; capillary blood testing 161; chaperoning 105, 106; confidentiality 56–57; Control of Substances Hazardous to Health (COSHH) regulations 98; disclosure 54; documentation 61; ear irrigation 258, 262; foot assessment 187; immunisation 228; lung function testing 215; venepuncture 151, 155; wound dressing 203; wound swabs 197
COPD *see* chronic obstructive pulmonary disease
cotton buds 257, 261
countersigning 62
COVID-19 239–240
criticism, coping with 50–51
cross-contamination 150
cultural differences 40, 41
curiosity 16
cyanosis 119
cycle of change 74, 80

dairy foods 77–78
Data Protection Act (2018) 53, 66
DBS (Disclosure and Barring Service) checks 104

dead space 210
debridement 198
decision-making 14
deep-vein thrombosis (DVT) 161
dehydration 163, 168, 169, 171
delegation 23, 24–27
dementia 42–43, 60, 70; communicating with a person with 44–46
depression 40, 82, 84, 205, 214
Deprivation of Liberty Safeguards (2009) 66
dermis 193–194
dextrocardia 146
diabetes 177–191; B_{12} deficiency 242; blood glucose 158–159; blood pressure 132; blood tests 156; common symptoms 190; diabetes insipidus 170; foot assessment 31; healthy eating 77; hyperlipidaemia 160; ketoacidosis 171; ketones 170; obesity 113; physical activity 82, 84; type 1 and type 2 177–179; urinalysis 169, 170; wound healing 205
Diabetes UK 177, 179, 182, 189
diaphragm 209–210
diaries, reflective 15
diarrhoea 170, 241, 243, 249
diastolic pressure 125, 126, 129
Di Clemente, C.C. 74
diet 76, 77, 79–81, 160, 171, 179, 242, 256
Different Health Boards and Trusts 68
digital documentation 62
dignity 7, 20, 42, 103, 105, 143, 203
disability 39, 67
disclosure 54–55
Disclosure and Barring Service (DBS) checks 104
distractions 40, 45
documentation: capillary blood testing 162; chaperoning 103; consent 58, 61; ear irrigation 262; ECG procedure 144; foot assessment 186, 187; immunisation 223; lung function testing 215; pulse oximetry 121; record-keeping 61–63; urinalysis 172; venepuncture 155; wound closures removal 205; wound dressing 204; wound swabs 197
domiciliary oxygen 214
Doppler 118, 184, 185
Down's syndrome 257

dressings 25–27, 197–204; antimicrobial 197; types of 198–200
Driscoll, J. 16
duty of care 23, 54, 65, 92, 229

ear anatomy 254–256
ear irrigation 24, 59, 253–265
earwax 253, 257, 259, 263, 264
echocardiography 135
e-cigarettes 85
eczema 200
Einthoven, W. 135
e-learning 75
electrocardiograph (ECG) 135
electrodes 141, 143, 144, 145
electrolytes 117, 157, 168
empathy 41
emphysema 213
empowerment 66
encephalitis 232
endocarditis 92
enzymes 150
epidemics 224, 230
epidermis 193
epithelialisation 195
erythrocyte sedimentation rate (ESR) 156
ethnicity 113
exacerbations 211
excoriation 198
exercise 82, 84; asthma 219; pulse rate 116; respiratory rate 119; urinalysis 169, 170
exfoliation 143
exudate 196, 197, 206
eye contact 39
eye damage 128, 158

facial expressions 36, 37, 45
fainting 117, 155
fat 76, 77, 113, 160, 178, 194, 245
fatigue 39–40, 158
fear 39–40
fever 121, 196, 235, 237, 249
fibre 77, 79
First Steps website 25
fistula 169
flu symptoms 225, 231, 234
flu vaccination 232–235, 244
foams 199
food 53–58, 59; *see also* diet
foot assessment 31, 187
forehead thermometers 122
fractional exhaled nitric oxide (FeNO) 212

Freedom of Information Act (2000) 53
fruit 77, 79
full blood count (FBC) 156
fungating wounds 199
fungi 92

gay patients 104
general practice (GP) contract 6
genitourinary tract 170
gestures 36, 37
Gibbs, G. 16, 17, 21
Gibbs' reflective cycle 16
Gillick Competency and Fraser
    Guidelines 59
glomerular filtration rate (GFR) 157
gloves 92, 95, 97–98, 152, 155, 202,
    203; capillary blood testing 161;
    ear irrigation 258; venepuncture
    152; wound care 197, 202
glucose 158–159; blood tests
    158–159; insulin resistance 113;
    kidney function 168; peripheral
    neuropathy 180; urinalysis 177
glycated/glycosylated haemoglobin see
    HbA1C
granulation 195
*The Green Book: Immunisation against
    Infection Disease* 223, 224
guidelines *see* protocols

haematuria 169
haemoglobin 156, 159
haemolysis 150, 151
haemophilia 149
haemostasis 194
hand hygiene 91, 93–95, 97, 98; hand-
    washing technique 95–97
HbA1C 159
HCAs *see* healthcare assistants
    (HCAs)
healing of wounds 194–195
health, definition of 73–75
healthcare assistants (HCAs) 1, 5–9
healthcare-associated infections
    (HCAIs) 92, 98
health care power of attorney 60
health promotion 73–86
healthy eating 76–79
heart anatomy 135–138
heart attack (myocardial infarction)
    113, 116, 117, 120, 128, 139, 140,
    141
heart disease 139–141; blood glucose
    158–159; blood tests 128;
    diabetes 177; healthy eating
    76–79; heart valve disease

161; hyperlipidaemia 160;
    hypertension 128; obesity 132;
    physical activity 82, 83; pulse rate
    117; risk factors 132; spirometry
    215–216; wound healing 205
heart failure 128, 140–141
heart rate 82, 116, 135, 138, 262
height measurement 114
hemosiderosis 183
heparin 161, 223
hepatitis 238
herd immunity 227
herpes zoster (shingles) 237–238
high-density lipoprotein (HDL) 132,
    160
Hippocratic oath 91
home blood pressure monitoring
    (HBPM) 126, 132
homocysteine 240
honest 37
honey 200
Hopi candling 263–264
hormones 126, 159, 168
HPV (human papilloma virus)
    vaccines 223
hydrocolloids 198
hydrofibre dressings 199
hydroxocobalamin 223, 242, 243
hypercoaguability 150
hyperlipidaemia 160; *see also*
    cholesterol; triglycerides
hyper-responsiveness 211
hypertension 126–127, 128;
    atherosclerosis 125; blood tests
    156; ECG procedure 141; healthy
    eating 76
hyperthermia 121
hyperthyroidism 116
hypotension 131
hypothermia 117, 121
hypoxia 117

immunisation/vaccines 60, 225–226;
    COVID-19 239–240; flu
    232–235; legal issues 228–230;
    pneumococcal 235–237; shingles
    (herpes zosters) 237–239;
    standards 224–225; storage
    227–228; types of 226–227
immunodeficiency 231
immunosuppression 150
inactivated/killed organisms 226
inborn immunity 225–226
infection 92–95, 196; chaperoning
    106; ear 253, 259; ECG procedure
    146; legislation and guidelines 98;

temperature measurement 121;
    urinalysis 168, 169; wounds 194,
    196, 201–202
inferior vena cava 137
inflammation 92, 156, 170, 211, 212
inflammatory bowel disease 242
influenza symptoms 231
influenza vaccination 59, 226, 230,
    232, 233
information: -gathering from the
    patient 35; use and protection
    of 66
informed consent *see* consent
inhalers 212–214, 217, 219
injections, administration of 223,
    228–230
inspections 29
insulin 113, 158, 177, 178
insulin resistance 113
insurance 25
intercostal recession 120
intercostal space 144, 145
international normalised ratio (INR)
    160–161
intestinal disease 158
intimate examinations 101–104
intramuscular (IM) injections 233,
    236, 243, 245–246, 248
intranasal vaccinations 228, 248–250
intravenous fluids 126
iodine 200
ischaemia 139, 184, 188

jargon 40, 62
Jasper, M. 14, 15
job description 1, 18, 23, 25
job satisfaction 35

Kessler, I. 5
ketoacidosis 169
ketones 170
kidney disease 126, 157, 158, 169, 236
kidney function 157, 167–173
kidney stones 158, 169
knowledge 1, 7, 24, 45, 149, 193, 229
Korotkoff sounds 129

language 40
learning 14
learning difficulties 39, 104
legal accountability 23
legal issues 228–230; administering
    injections 228–230;
    confidentiality 53–57; consent
    57–61; legal accountability 23;
    record-keeping 61–63

legislation 53, 54, 98–99
leucocytes 170
leukaemia 150
lipid profile test 160
listening 35, 39
live attenuated influenza vaccine (LAIV) 234–235
live attenuated vaccines 226
liver disease 80, 157, 158, 171
liver failure 171
liver function tests (LFTs) 157–158
loss of protective sensation (LOPS) 180, 185, 189, 190
low adherence 198
low-density lipoprotein (LDL) 132, 160
Ludwig, C. 125
lungs 209–220; BMI measurements 111; circulatory system 136; disease 210–212; function testing 214–218
lymph node clearance 152

maceration 198
Making Every Contact Count (MECC) 75
malaise 196, 235, 237
malignancy 111, 169
malnutrition 80, 111, 158
malpractice 101, 103
Medical Defence Union 103
Medical Protection 102, 103
medication: asthma 219; blood tests 157; hypertension 126; mucolytic 214; pulse oximetry 120; pulse rate 116; respiratory rate 119; shingles vaccination 238–239; urinalysis 171; wound healing 205
meningitis 232, 240
Mental Capacity Act (2005) 53, 61, 66
mental health 75, 85, 240
Mental Health Act (2007) 61
metabolic rate 80, 159
metabolism 119, 137, 160, 209
metformin 242
microorganisms 92, 93, 95, 196
Mid Staffordshire NHS Foundation Trust 7
mitral valve 137
MMR vaccine 224
monofilaments 184–185, 188, 189
monovette system 154
mRNA vaccines 227
MRSA 93
mucolytic medicines 214

myocardial infarction (heart attack) see heart attack (myocardial infarction)

National Institute for Health and Clinical Excellence (NICE) 29; asthma 210; blood pressure 132; BMI measurements 113; foot assessment 73; guidelines 29, 74; health promotion 73; infection control 98; National Minimum Standards and Core Curriculum for Immunisation Training of Healthcare Support Workers 223, 224, 229
National Occupational Standards: blood pressure measurement 129; capillary blood testing 161; delegation 24; ECG procedure 142; foot assessment 31; hand hygiene 95; physiological measurements 111; removal of wound closures 204; urinalysis 171; venepuncture 151; wound dressing 203
necrotic tissue 197
negligence 27, 33, 57, 58
nephrons 167, 168
neurological (nerve) disease 158
NHS and Community Care Act (1990) 5
NHS Choices 97, 241
NHS & Community Care Act (1990) 5
NHS Confidentiality Code of Practice (2003) 53
NHS England 75, 99, 209
NICE see National Institute for Health and Clinical Excellence
nicotine replacement therapy 85, 86
nitrites 170
NMC see Nursing and Midwifery Council
non-verbal communication 37–39
Nursing and Midwifery Council (NMC) 7, 8, 24
nursing apprentice 9
nursing associate (NA) 8, 9
nursing auxiliaries 5

obesity 77, 79; alcohol 80; body mass index 112, 113; classification 112; diabetes 179; high blood pressure 132; risk assessment with waist measurement 113
odour-absorbent dressings 199
Oelofsen, N. 16, 21

older people: blood pressure 126; earwax treatment 257; flu vaccination 232, 233; physical activity 83; pneumococcal vaccination 236; shingles 238
olive oil 257
omega-3 77
opiate analgesics 120
oral digital thermometers 122
orthostatic proteinuria 169
osteoporosis 111
otitis media 232, 235
overfamiliarity 41
oxygen 119, 120, 156; anaemia 240; breathing 119, 209–210; domiciliary 214; pulse oximetry 120; wound healing 195

pain 35, 39–40, 139, 237, 238, 242, 259
palliative care 214
pandemics 230
paraffin gauze 199
parental responsibility 60
partnership 66
passive immunity 226
Pasteur, L. 91
pathogens 92, 93, 196, 226, 227
patient group directions (PGDs) 228
Patient.info 74, 77, 79, 80
patient satisfaction 35
patient-specific directions (PSDs) 219, 223, 228–230, 235, 243
peak flow recording 214–215, 218
pericardial tamponade 116
peripheral neuropathy 179, 180–181, 242
peripheral vascular disease 128, 181
personality clashes 40
personal protective equipment (PPE) 91, 92, 98, 99, 202, 262
pH 171
phlebotomy 6, 149; see also venepuncture
physical activity 81–84; see also exercise
platelet function disorders 150
platelets 149, 150, 156, 194
Pneumococcal disease 235–236
pneumococcal pneumonia 223, 227
Pneumococcal polysaccharide vaccine (PPV23) 236
pneumonia 92, 223, 227, 235, 238, 239
pneumothorax 220
polycythaemia 126
population immunity 227
post-herpetic neuralgia (PHN) 238

postural hypotension 130–131
posture 37
potassium 150, 157, 168, 171
power of attorney 60
PQRST 135, 138–139
pre-eclampsia 169
pregnancy: avoidance of alcohol during 67–68; dressings 200; healthy eating 76–77; influenza vulnerability 230–231; spirometry 215–216; urinalysis 169; vaccinations 231, 235, 236
privacy 7, 20, 105–106, 143
Prochaska, J. O. 74
professional accountability 23
protein 77, 79, 157, 169, 227
protocols 25, 29–33; purpose of 29–30; template 31–32; working without 33
Public Health England (PHE) 75, 76, 82, 224
public interest 54
pulmonary embolism 161
pulse amplitude 117
pulse measurement 116–117
pulse oximetry 120–121
pulse pressure 126
pyelonephritis 170
pyrexia 116, 121, 169, 196, 234, 235

RCN see Royal College of Nursing
recombinant vaccines 227
record-keeping 61–63
rectal thermometers 122
red blood cells 126, 150, 156, 159, 163, 168, 171, 240
reflection 13–21; example 17–21; frameworks for 16–17; practice 14; stages 16; writing 14, 15–16
reflective cycle 16
REFLECT model 17
regulation 6–7
renal artery stenosis 168, 171
renal dialysis 163
renal function tests (RFTs) 157
reperfusion 184
resident flora 93
residual volume 210
respect 40
respiratory disease 209, 212, 235; see also chronic obstructive pulmonary disease
respiratory rate 119–120
responsibility 23
reversibility testing 217, 218–220

'ride your green bike' (RYGB) mnemonic 145
rights 19, 20, 47, 48, 51
risk: delegation 24; ear irrigation 258, 259, 262; public interest disclosure 54; ulceration 182, 187–188; warning of 58
Riva-Rocci, S. 125
Rotherham Ear Centre 253, 261, 262
Royal College of Nursing (RCN) 5; First Steps website 25; immunisation 243; protocols 30

safeguarding 65–70; HCA role 67–70; history of 65–66; persons at risk 67
safety 146, 223
salbutamol 116, 212, 213, 219
salt 77–78, 167
Savile, J. 101
scales 114
self-esteem 51
'sensitive' examinations 103–104; see also intimate examinations
sharps 91, 92, 99, 153, 154, 204
shingles 223, 237–239
Shingrix 227, 239
Shipman, H. 101
sick sinus syndrome 116
silver dressings 199
sinus/sino-atrial (SA) node 138, 140
skills 25, 47
Skills for Care/Skills for Health codes of conduct 7
skin 193–206; healthy eating 76; skin anatomy 193–194; temperature measurement 183; wound care 193–206; wound healing 194–195
slough 194, 197
smoking 75, 84–86, 170, 213; asthma 213; atherosclerosis 181; COPD 213–214; diabetes 179; wound healing 205
social media 56
sodium 157, 168, 257
specific gravity (SG) 170
spirometry 209, 212, 215–219
state-enrolled nurses (SENs) 5
statins 158
steroids 212, 213
stimulants 116
stress 102, 119, 139
stroke: atrial fibrillation 140; blood glucose 158; healthy eating 77, 78; homocysteine 240; hyperlipidaemia 160;

hypertension 128; venepuncture 152; warfarin 161
subcutaneous fat 194
subcutaneous (SC) injections 247–248
sugar 76, 79
superior vena cava 137
supervision 24
support 224 24
surgical site infection 98
surgical wounds 121; see also wound care
sutures 204
swabbing 196–197, 201
systolic pressure 125

tachycardia 116
telephone confidentiality 56
temperature measurement 121–123
thermometers 122
thyroid disease 158, 160
thyroid function tests 159
tidal breathing 210
total lung capacity 210
touch 41, 93
tourniquets 151–155, 244
trachea 210
trainee nursing associate (TNA) 8, 9
training 6, 7, 23, 31; ear irrigation 253; immunisation 223–225; lung function testing 216; protocols 31; wound care 193
transformation 17
transgender patients 104
transient flora 93
tricuspid valve 137
triglycerides 132, 160
tuning forks 189
turbid 168
tympanic thermometers 122

ulceration 187–188
ultra-processed food (UPF) 78
updates 25
urea 157
urinalysis 167–173

vaccination see immunization/ vaccines
vacuette system 152, 153
vagus nerve 262
varicose eczema 200
varicose veins 183
vascular access devices 98
vegetables 77
veins 135, 137, 151; collapsed 155; palpable 151, 152; varicose 183

venepuncture 57, 59, 149–164
venuoles 137
verbal communication 37
verbal consent 58, 151
VibraTip 188–189
vicarious liability 27, 33
viruses 92, 98, 196, 226, 230, 231
vitamin B_{12} *see* B_{12} deficiency
vitamin D 84, 194, 223
vitamin K 149, 157, 161

waist measurement 111–113
warfarin 160–161
waste disposal 98
wax 253, 256–257, 259–262
weight loss 80, 179
weight measurement 114–116
white blood cells 156, 170, 194
World Health Organization (WHO) 67, 73, 232
wound care 193–206; *see also* dressings

wound closures, removal of 204–206
wound dressing *see* dressings
wound healing 194–196
writing, reflective 15–16
written consent 59

zinc paste bandages 200
Zostavax 238, 239
Z-track technique 246

Printed in the United States
by Baker & Taylor Publisher Services